Suddenly Terminal

Sharon Dawson

SUDDENLY TERMINAL

ISBN:9798432157201

SUDDENLY TERMINAL

CONTENTS

SUDDENLY TERMINAL

CONTENTS

SUDDENLY TERMINAL

For Tommy and for Brandon.

Without your loyalty, devotion, patience, tears, joy and belief in me, I simply would not have survived.

ACKNOWLEDGMENTS

This book was born when I was dying. Kind of Ironic, eh? And, as always, it takes a village to help with the care and handling of me.

Therefore, I need to acknowledge the villagers who have made this book happen, not to mention my life.

It seems only fitting that we start with my life, doesn't it? That would be my medical team, starting with my oncologist, Dr. Mark Turrill, MD and his terrific team of nurses and staff including the office staff who patiently fielded neurotic phone calls from me more times than I care to admit to. Every nurse in the place is wonderful, but two in particular. One is Rosa Sander, RN whose even temperament and demeaner is instantly calming. Her gentle laugh and humor is a huge calming force for everyone in the Infusion Room. She *emits* a sense of safety. The second one is Kerrylea O'Brien, RN. I really do not have words to tell you what a lifeline this woman has been to me through all my treatments. She is calming and reassuring, like Rosa, but beyond that she notices every detail she can about every individual patient. I always knew that she knew who I was and wanted to know more. She genuinely cared. Aside from literally saving my life when I went into whatever reaction thing I had, she saved me on other levels as well. She seemed to have a grasp on who I was and a gift for reminding me of that. I never felt like she saw me as "another cancer patient". She only saw me as Sharon.

And to my actual village. I live in a tiny little town and I've blessed with phenomenal kindness and thoughtfulness throughout this whole ordeal. Little gifts would make their way to me, gestures of caring. And while I remained in isolation, those served to remind me that there are very good people out there rooting for me. It meant more than I can tell you. Thank you all for that and for respecting my privacy while I healed and came back to life.

But my village extends far beyond the borders of this town; it extends to my fantastic on-line community that has diligently read every word I wrote about this and encouraged me keep writing and to write a book. It has taken a great deal of courage to do, being as it is so personal, but it is all of you who gave me the strength to go for it. So I thank you.

Writing a book is no small task, let me tell you. Even one this small can be almost overwhelming and confusing. Then when you are "done" (the first time you think you are done, anyway) – you re-read and find a myriad of things wrong with it. This is where editors and proof readers come in. Their job is to keep me from public humiliation! They say a second set of eyes is a good idea. I think eight extra eyes is what it took for me! So, to my dear friends, Laura Trovillion, Mary Dearing, Jenifer Popovich, and John Sullivan – My love and complete gratitude. You are unexpected angels and likely the bravest people I know. (Definitely the most *tolerant* people I know!)

I love all of you,
Sharon

INTRODUCTION

In 2016, I finally dragged my ass in to get a long overdue mammogram. It turned out I had a little space alien in my right boob. I was shocked, terrified, and *sure* I was going to die. I cried all the time, scared to death. But Terminal was never really there. Hypochondria and Over Imagination were definitely there but not Terminal. The other two are easily assuaged by friends. My *Fear* of Terminal was there in, but *he, himself,* wasn't.

Stage one lump was removed by a partial mastectomy. I pretty much cruised through the surgery, and my oncologist informed me that I did NOT have to do chemo, but that three weeks of radiation was a good idea.

The deal with radiation is that it is a daily gig. In order to do this, and keep my same doctor, whom I liked, would mean driving an hour and a half each way, every day, for three weeks. If I switched to another provider it would only be a half hour each way. Being ignorant enough to still think that all oncologists are created equal, I switched doctors. I did the radiation and was given a pill called anastrozole that I was to take for the following five years. About

18 months into it, I began to get suspicious. Something had changed. Not only in my body, but in my doctor's approach to things. Suddenly, I was getting random tests that didn't seem to have a damn thing to do with my boobs. Upon questioning my doctor, I learned that he was an arrogant demigod who had zero respect for me as a person and was incapable, and/or unwilling, to discuss this with me.

Everything in my body told me to get off these damn pills. He was insistent that if I did that, I would immediately get my breast cancer back. So I kept taking them. *I shouldn't have.*

Six months later, I got my period at age 59. Turns out that endometrial cancer is a rare side effect of this stupid pill, and that is what it was.

Suffice it to say that I fired him and returned to my original doctor. One hysterectomy and six months later, I had a scan and was given the "all clear".

About six months after *that*, I started to feel pretty tired. Naps were a new norm for me, but hey! I'm not as young as I used to be, *right*? As time went on, I got more and more tired. It was a particularly hot summer so I blamed it on *that*. (Never mind my central air conditioning and the days where I couldn't get off the couch *at all*; denial is a beautiful thing.) I just needed more exercise, *right*? I would lie on the couch and vow to join the gym. *Every day.*

By mid-July my stomach was definitely growing. This I passed off as getting older, always having been a stomach person, drinking wine and *still* not exercising. I also blamed it on being married to a chef who is addicted to potato chips and *very* generous with the latter.

At this point, I found myself having a rapid heartbeat from time to time. While I attempted to throw this onto my pile of excuses, I decided it might be time for me to see my doctor. This would be my general practitioner, not my oncologist. This doctor's MO is to pass people off to his PA whenever possible, but I really wanted to see *him. Something was going on.* His first available appointment was a month later.

That month began the acceleration into Hell. My stomach blew up, like I was nine months pregnant. I hurt *everywhere.* Sitting was almost impossible. I fell and broke a rib. We all got sick. I fell again. And again. My legs were no longer dependable. I grew very weak. Swallowing became difficult. I began to throw up. Eating was almost impossible. I ceased to have regular bowel movements. Finally, I was at the doctor's office.

While I could count the number of meals I had eaten in the last three weeks on one hand, I had still managed to gain ten pounds. *Something was very, very wrong.*

I'm going to spare you the ludicrous futility of that appointment except to say he determined that I was *constipated.* I was sent to the pharmacy to purchase every over-the-counter medication that they make, including enemas.

Nothing worked. I kept getting worse and worse and *worse.* The puking accelerated. I started bleeding rectally. I continually called my doctor, to no avail.

Five days later, it was my 61st birthday. A Saturday. A few close friends came over. They had been watching this digression and when I could eat nothing but a little watermelon, they and my family decided I needed to go to the ER *right then.* I refused with good reason. In order to sit for dinner, I was in a wheelchair with a back brace made for a much smaller person, and five pillows. That made the pain just bearable enough to do it. No way in *hell* was I going to spend hours in a waiting room chair on a Saturday night.

They went home. I threw up all over the place (bile, no food in me but two bites of watermelon). My husband, Tommy, gave me a codeine and helped me get into bed.

In the morning my friend Rachel showed up and duly announced that I was either getting in the car and going *willingly* with her to the ER or she was calling 911. Much as I wanted to believe the constipation diagnosis, I knew something much worse was to blame. I went.

Everyone was pleasant (except me). Changing into the gown from hell (Seriously? We can put a man on the moon but we can't develop something beyond a Rubik's Cube for a hospital gown?), trying to even lay down without help, never mind getting *on* the bed, telling people my birthdate every six seconds without puking, all under horrific fluorescent lights, was not conducive to my natural demeanor. But I tried. The ER doc came in, all business, checked some things, actually *looked* at my stomach (something my GP failed to do) and – here's a concept – he also looked at my *chart*. (Something my GP *also* failed to do.)

"You had a hysterectomy due to endometrial cancer a little over a year ago, right?"

Next thing I knew I was being marched off to X-ray and to get a CT scan. It's a Sunday so the people who read the CT scans aren't there and the doctor tells me they have to find someone to do it. He also told me that it was decidedly NOT constipation and to stop with all the stool softeners, etc. He wanted to know who told me I was constipated. When I told him it was my GP, he wanted to know his name. He then disappeared for what seemed like hours. I called Rachel to tell her to go home and I would call her when I was done. She refused.

This was making me very nervous. I decided it was probably gastritis.

When the ER doc came back in, he was clearly upset. He sat down in front of me as I sat on the bed and told me that he had news and it wasn't good.

"Yup", I'm thinking, "Gastritis."

Then he asked me if my "sister" (I had lied in a failed attempt to get Rachel in there with me) was still there. I said yes.

"The news I have for you is bad. It's *really* bad. Do you want me to get her? I think you should have someone with you." He had tears in his eyes. That didn't bode well.

He went to get her and I spent the longest five minutes of my life waiting. So much for my gastritis plan.

When they came back in, I could see that Rachel was very unnerved as well. Doctors do not come get you out of a car in the parking lot. That really doesn't happen.

He sat back down in front of me and I heard his voice breaking.

"This is not constipation. One look at your chart told me that. Your endometrial cancer has returned and has spread throughout your body. This should be obvious to any medical professional. The bloating in your stomach is caused by this cancer. You need to have a paracentesis done. This is where they drain the fluid out of you. You are neither a candidate for surgery nor radiation. There is a *chance* that you still might be able to get chemotherapy. You need to contact an oncologist right away. This is very aggressive and it is spreading *very* fast."

He looked miserable and my heart went out to him. I was in shock.

"How long?"

"Without treatment? Two to four months max."

So much for being cancer-free! I listened to a few more things. Rachel saw right away that I was absorbing *none* of it and took over with the questions. I don't remember any of that part. Just that I decided I needed to go home. *Right then.*

I announced that I was leaving and anything further could be discussed freely with my "sister" and she could sign anything needed. I threw on my jeans and sweater, over my gown, grabbed the car keys and went to the car.

I simply could not be there anymore. She found me chain-smoking in the car. Ironically my x-ray showed my lungs were clear. Besides, four months? *Why the hell not?*

I don't remember the drive home much. I remember her telling me I needed to quit smoking and, after one murderous look from yours truly, amended with, "but maybe not *today*." Pretty sure I cried, pretty sure we both said, "fuck" a lot, but I really don't know.

Tommy was home when I got there. My youngest son, Brandon, was also. I don't remember telling them. I don't remember much else from that day. I know I wanted to call my Mom more than anything. But then I remembered that she already knew. She had died the year before. I know I called my sisters and my older son, Collin. Rachel cleaned my kitchen and told Tommy everything she could about the appointment and went home to fall apart alone

I simply went *numb*.

1. NOTHING

Nothing. I feel exactly nothing. It's like a big sign that reads N.O.T.H.I.N.G. sitting on top of me as I lay in the dark. I ponder this for a moment. No obnoxious twinges. Bladder uninvolved. Yep. *Nothing.* And my brain is quiet. I am liking Nothing. I'm *afraid* to move. I know the second I move Something is going to come on the scene and Something is likely going to *hurt.*

I just want to enjoy Nothing some more. I'm reveling in Nothing. I simply lie there. I want to take in every moment of this because I know all too well it is short lived. And I have Silence too, I realize. THAT is a rarity around here. Everybody is still asleep (which is not a rarity) and nobody, including all three dogs AND my husband, are snoring. (THAT is most *decidedly* a rarity). When cancer gets on the stage of your life, it isn't often you get to feel NOTHING, and most certainly not with the added bonus of Silence. There are lots of Somethings to feel and you feel them in degrees.

I *love* my bed. We have had this bed for almost five years. I couldn't wait to have it. We had lost our house in one of the now-constant California wildfires and were staying in my mother-in-law's basement while we rebuilt. We were sleeping on a slab of concrete cleverly *disguised* as a bed. We were grateful for what we had, no doubt about that, but we woke to crippled hips every morning and shoulders to match. Then one day they finished building our new house and we slept on our new bed. We learned to truly appreciate things. Just like I am appreciating Nothing right now. Is Nothing a Something that having cancer is teaching me to appreciate? I guess so. But I don't want to think about that right now. The word Terminal is too new, too sudden, and I'm going to have to take that one on slowly.

Every. Single. Night. I appreciate my bed. I have a double pillowtop CA King, and soft, squishy down pillows (I've never understood people who like to sleep on firm pillows. I find it more akin to a wrestling match with SpongeBob SquarePants than anything *remotely* close to comfortable). I have perfectly crisp, Egyptian Cotton white sheets and a 100% down comforter. None of that down/feather bullshit where the evil little feathers wiggle out to stab you. I smile. The fire turned me into a bed snob, apparently. But I *appreciate* what I have. Like my friend Nothing here.

My Brain begins to review the upcoming day. These days it has much to do with what I'm going to watch on Netflix when I have to hit the nest, formally known as the couch. I wonder what time it is. That's the trouble with being an early riser at this time of year. I get up and it could be 3 AM (not good) or it may be 5 AM which is OK.

It's time to say Goodbye to Nothing for the moment. I send it along with a little package of Gratitude to take with it, and move into Something.

I have Cancer. Oh boy. Now *that's* Something.

2. TERMINAL

All the doors were locked in my mind. I couldn't take any more information right then. I just needed quiet, I wanted to absorb my diagnosis for a minute. Then I heard breaking windows. I guess denial is no match for this particular burglar, here to invade my thoughts and my life. His name is Terminal and apparently, he is moving in.

Also apparently I now have the Ultimate Unwanted Houseguest, who doesn't seem to *care* that he is unwanted and the word "guest" is something I attach, clinging to the part of me that believes in miracles.

I have met Terminal before. But under entirely different circumstances. I've had a couple goes with cancer prior to this, and Terminal loves to take you on a practice run at times like that. You cry a lot. But he's not *really* there. You can't *see* him. I guess those instances are more built around the *fear* of Terminal than Terminal *himself*. And I've watched him set up shop for a few of my dearly beloved, but I'm learning that when he arrives on YOUR scene it's entirely *something else altogether*.

When I first spotted him, I thought, "You have to be kidding me! This is IT?". I guess I had been expecting to see some villainous, evil, tall, dark old man with snaggle teeth and a hateful sneer. You know the guy – think Snape in the Harry Potter series. But nooooo. Not *this* guy. First of all, he's short. Very short. And young. Maybe 30? His hair is a tasseled mop of blond and he's sporting blue jeans, some old suit coat and bare feet. He's bright eyed and has some sort of beret-type hat going on. Great. I get a cross between a hippie and a wanna-be golfer. Admittedly, I was rather taken aback by this.

And…It seems that he is moving in. The first thing he does is clear out part of my brain to make room for himself. Apparently, my filter is a *problem* for Terminal, who has locked up what's left of my filter in a cupboard. My verbal filter was very decrepit to start with, but at least he was THERE! Now he is *gone* and has seemingly been replaced with an I-Don't-Care- Attitude. I'm still an inherently polite person, thank God, or jail might be next for throttling one of the How-Can-I-Make-Your-Cancer-All-About-Me Gang. There's everybody's big dream! Incarcerated and dying! I think I really need what is left of my filter.

I ask, "Just, exactly, WHAT do you think you are doing by locking up parts of me without my express permission?"
"Oh, get over it," he says, waving me off in an entirely-too-casual-for-me kind of way, "It's about time for him to retire anyway. Just listen to him, for Pete's sake! Does that sound like a working filter to you?"

He does have a point. The string of creative swear words coming out of the cupboard at that moment were decidedly NOT filtered.

"I am not sure this is such a great idea, to be honest."
"'Honest' is the key word here, Sharon. You have to be honest right now. Brutally honest. You know already that you have no energy to give anyone else. You barely have enough to give yourself and some people, not everyone, but some people are inherently prone to making everything about themselves. They are going to require too much energy from you now. You are angry."

"Damn straight, you little invasive rodent! I'm not happy with you at all!"
The big dramatic sigh that came out of him was followed with an overly-patient and condescending tone (which I later learned was Terminal at his wit's end), "Of course you are angry at me. Can't say that is an unusual response to my arrival, sadly. But what I am talking about here is the part where you have a propensity to put yourself last and you can't do that now. Besides, there are going to be some people who will really let you down. And if you can't be honest about what you need, unfiltered, then that isn't fair when someone fails your unspoken expectations, is it? I'm appealing to your COMPASSIONATE nature." The last was said without the patient tone and laced with sheer sarcasm.

Obviously I had a multi-*faceted* house guest. This was going to be interesting.

But he had a point. Right out of the gate I had become irritated with a few people who really let me down. Just a few, but they let me down *badly*. Some people were just too much for me - period. Some people that I had expectations of simply disappeared on both myself *and* my husband, and some people just made a simple misstep in conversation and I jumped on them like a crazed tiger. THAT last issue is why I needed my filter, I duly pointed this out to Terminal.

"No you don't. First of all, your filter needs to go into the shop for some serious repair. If you take a good, hard look at how it's been working for you in the last few years, you should see that it wasn't doing the best of jobs. Particularly in a few instances where you secretly didn't like the person in the first place. You have to work on DISCRIMINATION kiddo. THAT is what you need. And you need to put that stuff out there unfiltered. I'm telling you that you will save yourself a lot of grief in the future."
"I have a FUTURE?"
Exasperated, he answers, "Yes, you have a FUTURE. Next week can be considered the future for that matter. What you seemingly DON'T have are EARS!!!"
I'm sure he's right about the ear thing because all I can hear is

that I only have next week. And believe me, my rapidly disintegrating body is in full agreement. "I guess the word 'future' is relative?"

Ignoring this, he says, "THE second thing about removing your filter, and why it is in such bad need of repair, is you need to be honest with YOURSELF! You lie to yourself! You have more paranoias and phobias and bullshit going through your head for the sole sake of being 'loved' and accepted by anyone except YOURSELF! And in regards to your future and how long you have- that is up to you, ultimately. I am here to help you live whatever life you have left to the fullest, if you want me to. But that choice is going to have to be yours. You will be happy to know that you are, ultimately, in control. So, do you want me to let your filter out, or can I clean this damn place up first?"

"Fine. Do what you do. I'm willing to acquiesce the point. For the moment. It's a lot to think about."

"I know you are hurt. And one day you will get your filter back, I promise you. And one day the people who can't handle you right now may come back. But you might be surprised how you feel about that when it happens. You know that old saying, 'You don't know what you've got 'till it's gone'? Well, just wait and see how you feel about it when it comes back."

I stood there for a minute. I didn't get it right away. I don't know if I'm being terribly naive, dense or just stubborn, "So, you are saying that these people will show up at the end and I will be super happy to see them? 'Cuz I'm kinda pissed right now. Really pissed, as a matter of fact."

"Oh for fuck's sake, Sharon! What I am saying is that when you get your newly repaired filter back with its upgrade of discrimination, you may decide then, with clearer eyes, if you even WANT these people back in your life. You are a mess right now. There is no way in hell you can figure it out. Stop worrying about other people and just do what you need to do. I'm here because you are DYING! You have a limited time to live. Do you get that? Don't live it for others, live it for YOURSELF!"

And there it was. Right in front of me. The simple truth - I was going to *die*. And here I was, clinging to what I had considered "normal", angry at a small handful of people who were failing me.

Failing me *how*, exactly? By not calling me? By wanting to divert the highly uncomfortable situation into their own problems, which I suddenly considered unimportant and petty where I had always been compassionate before? And now I was *angry* about that? Terminal was right. I needed to be honest with myself and everybody around me. I was being very unfair, but I couldn't help it.

It was too much to think about anymore. I took a pain pill, went to bed and vowed to myself that I would try to understand and learn. Even if the future *was* only a week long; I was going to live that week more honestly.

We didn't have much to do with each other for a few days. Frankly, I was trying to ignore him. He's hard to ignore, however.

He's been busy with his room in my brain. He sweeps a lot and occasionally I hear a few scuffles as he has put something other than the cobwebs in the trash bin. Despite his resistance, I have insisted on looking through what he's throwing out. Most of it I completely agreed with. One of the first things I spotted was a pile of old jeans that didn't fit me. I was confused at first until I realized he was trying to get rid of superfluous crap that I have and don't need, like old jeans that no longer fit me. I HATE these jeans. They are uncomfortable critters that one feels socially obligated to wear because one lives in a society where Cute Butt is paramount. I was given Flat Butt, though. Getting rid of material clutter that does not make me feel good about myself is a *great* idea. I sanctioned that plan and I was given a pat on the back. I don't know if I actually like this guy, but he sure is *interesting*. And he is giving me something to think about besides imminent death (my body was busily reminding me of that on its own.)

But sometimes I don't like him *one little bit*. He's pushy, domineering, and oftentimes completely out of line. It's times like this that we get into a bit of a row about things. One instance was in regards to my Overly-Empathetic Camp Counselor persona. I've long been the polite, caring and compassionate person who people can lay their troubles on. I didn't want to give that up. That was *me!* It was an inherent part of my career, my persona, and at the forefront of my interpersonal relationships. I left him scowling and went downstairs to go about other things. I only give Terminal so much of my time in a day and he has been admonished to spend the rest in his own quarters. Therefore, I was surprised when he showed up in my personal space, off hours, and started rummaging around for my ever-elusive Windex. He announced that he was washing my windows; they were filthy.

A few days later he asked me to come up and See. There were a lot of crystal-clear windows. All bright and sparkly. Most of them showed beautiful scenes of nature, but one showed a steep, uphill, rocky path and I saw myself, much akin to a momma dog with ten pups attached to her teats, slowly trying to traverse this path with this huge burden attached. I was very sad at first because I knew then that most of those pups did not have the ability to emotionally reciprocate and help carry the load. It's as though they wanted to get their very last few drops of breast milk in, even if it only meant exhausting and depleting Momma's remaining energy. I tentatively gave Terminal permission to throw out the Camp Counselor routine.

"Good for you. It's your turn now."

I thought that only happened on birthdays. Quick! Someone hand me a balloon!

I went downstairs and absorbed this for a bit. The next day I announced my retirement and closed my studio. It didn't make me too sad. I have long dreamed of retiring and focusing the last chapter of my life on writing. Albeit sooner than I had thought and a much *shorter* last chapter than I anticipated, mercifully I still had one. Terminal has given me a break for now. He's got his room all sorted (I'm still working on mine) and I see that his mission has been to help me with MY mission which is to enjoy what's *left* of my life. He is helping me reduce the perpetual mental clutter. I'm not done, and I know it, but happiness has some room around here now, and like they say: One Step at a Time.

3. THE MATE

Many people have the great misfortune of going through this alone. I'm *very* grateful not to be one of those people. Even without a spouse, most of us are blessed with somebody, a friend, a child, clergy, SOMEBODY. If you don't have a soul, look for a support group. Try, anyway.

"And there is always me – don't forget – I'm here too!" Terminal yells from his room.
"Oh yes – YOU! The ever unwelcome and ever-present Diagnosis From Hell. Yessiree Bob!– just what everyone is looking for! You nailed it Terminal – right on the head. Pretty sure most people would pick Alone over your ass. Just sayin'...

He shut up then so I could think and reflect without him.

I happen to be blessed in my later years with an incredible husband. (After an embarrassing and excessive amount of frog kissing.) The second I was given my diagnosis he was *all in.* He took a leave of absence and we started, blindly, to traverse this path. Both of us were terrified, but we were *together.*

I had been disintegrating with the-cancer-I-didn't-know-I-had for at least a couple months when I got the actual diagnosis. Mostly it was my increasing stomach weight and back pain. We tried our level best to manage it ourselves. Back braces, strategic pillows, on and on. I kept trying to be the same person I was before. Little by little, that became less and less possible.

When I returned home with my diagnosis and, albeit unwittingly, Terminal in tow, it was a bombshell and a half. While we all knew something was very wrong, I don't think any of us were ready for *this*.

In that moment and in the days that followed, I saw all of my dreams crashing down around me. And I saw the same thing happening to my husband. The guilt was overwhelming; worse than anything else, I think. Here is this hard-working, loyal, and lovely man, whose dreams are shattered because of me. I knew that there was nothing I could do; that this wasn't of my own making, but that didn't *change* anything. *My* CANCER was taking hostages. He had just gotten robbed of his dreams and plans and, bottom line, no matter how you slice it, it was all on account of me.

I tried to hide my feelings and put on a happy face the best I could, but it didn't work for long. My pain was very obvious and the more independent I tried to be (which was an absolute joke at that point) the more useless and helpless he felt. Nothing I could do would make it better. We were both lost in the face of this monster.

I fought my whole life to be independent on every level. I've been through some serious shit in my day. Abandonment issues and all that jazz. Like everyone, I secretly wanted to find that one person who would really love me. However, I was convinced that I was ultimately unlovable and would subsequently be abandoned again. Sooooo... I figured that if I had autonomy in my profession and, on some level, my personal life, it wouldn't kill me when they inevitably left me.

Over our 15 years together, Tommy has shown me that I *can* trust him. That we were partners in the truest sense as far as he was concerned.

Clearly metastatic cancer calls for retirement. I could be wrong, but after 40 years as a professional photographer, I felt pretty sure that in order to do my job, I would need to pick *up* the camera which I couldn't physically do. So I closed my studio. My new job was to stay alive.

Suddenly I hear the Bee Gees *blasting* from the other room "Whether you're a brother or whether you're a mother you're stayin' alive…. Ah, ha, ha, ha Stayin' Aliiiiive……"

Dear God. "TERMINAL!!?!" The thumping stops and the music cuts.
"WHAT?"
"Is this REALLY necessary? I'm on a train of thought here and this is not helping!"
"I love that song! Are you sure it isn't helping?"
"Pretty damn sure, yes. If you can't stay OUT of what I'm doing here, will you at least TRY to keep quiet?"
"Maybe".

As I am pretty sure that this is the best I'm going to get from him; I continue to write.

Tommy took over handling all of my bills at that point. That was hard for me. I like control and I don't like having to justify how and when I spend my money. I was dead sure that this was going to happen, but, to my surprise, it didn't. This was amazing to me. And to have someone take that stress off of me and do it WELL was a downright shock to my system (particularly the latter because, if the truth be told, While I've *managed* to do it, but I've never managed to do it *well*).

It was good for me, in retrospect. ….

"RETROSPECT! Do you hear yourself?"
"I'm TRYING to hear myself, but it's a little difficult."

"Retrospect – get it? You didn't think you were going to live to this point, much less be able to look at something in 'retrospect'". Then he busted out the Stayin' Alive song again.

Wow. He had a point.

But nothing really mattered much then. Most of my motivation was due to an unspoken awareness that I was going to die *quite* soon and I didn't want to leave Tommy mystified as to what was going on in the other half of our personal finances. I made light of this fact as much as I could so as not to become maudlin. That would hurt him far and away too much and I couldn't bear the thought of that.

My physical decline was accelerating rapidly. And I mean *rapidly*. While I was miserable even then, I didn't believe the doctor completely about the two to four months thing on Diagnosis Day. But within a few weeks, I not only *believed* it, but I was pretty sure it would be the shorter end of the stick. While I tried to hide this as much as I could from my loved ones, once it began to physically manifest, it became impossible to hide.

Wheelchairs, for instance, are both blatant and obvious. So are portable toilets in the living room. So is the part where I couldn't get *to* the toilet, never mind get *on* the toilet and just forget about getting *off* the damn thing. I would probably still be there had it not been for Tommy and Brandon.

I was damn near helpless. The pain was constant, varying only in degrees; never going away. To roll over in bed involved help and it still hurt like hell. Sitting in the car was almost unbearable, never mind *getting to* the car, and *driving? Not an option.* Simply not an option.

Since I couldn't do much about the screaming or grimacing (pain is pain), I hid the tears as much as I could. I knew that every tear was a knife in Tommy's heart.

That part is tricky. That part is *very* tricky. It is the double-edged sword from Hell, actually. Clearly the motivation is to protect the ones we love most. But that is rather silly when you think about it – they are already affected and I wasn't hiding anything physically. But I was hiding my fear from them as much as I could. I knew if they fell I had nothing left to help them get up. And beyond that – if *they* fell down, there would be no way *I* could get up.

Not too many years ago, my best friend of 40+ years was suddenly diagnosed with brain cancer and given a year to live. She fought long and hard and made it almost five years. In 2017, I was diagnosed with breast cancer and I hit Terrified at MACH III force. I asked her. I asked her how in the hell she handled it. She said, "You cry a lot the first year. Then you stop and it simply becomes part of who you are." We cried together many times. I hold that dear to me; not the crying, per se, but the words.

I've stayed friends with her husband, and we talk from time to time. Just the other day he told me that she had also told him that. Then he said, "Sharon? I never once saw her cry."

For him that was hard. He had been a mind-boggling caretaker for her and she was, and always will be, his soul-mate. He took it as a failure on his part. I, however, now being on this side of things, fully understood. So, I explained it to him. It was a sign of her deep love for him and her trying to protect him. I think it helped; at least I *hope* it did.

I am also *afraid* to start crying. Everybody thinks I am so strong. Maybe I am, but I am not strong enough to risk taking myself and everyone else I love down into my depression. I know if I cry, I will not be able to stop. I'm going to focus on staying alive, and just not jump into that deep, dark well below my feet. One tear would push me over the edge, I'm sure of it.

"Can I sing now?"
"NO!"

I've been on the "other side of the fence" an awful lot. It's different, but it is probably equally painful to watch your beloved

19

dying. Add to that not wanting to upset each other with your own fears, and you are both left in limbo. When the person you counted on the most to be able to talk to can't talk to *you* because they don't want to hurt you and vice-versa, it does not bode well for the relationship.

Mercifully, my life travels have shown me the beauty of hospice. Now, don't freak out at the word. I'm not saying you need to trot right out of the doctor's office and straight into hospice. *Not at all.* What I *am* saying is that they offer a wonderful bereavement service to EVERYONE. And you do not need to be receiving their services otherwise, signed up or actively dying. And it is *free*. Free counseling that focuses on the situation at hand and how to cope with it, not trying to dive into your fourth year on the planet and what the creepy neighbor was doing in bed with your sister. I have used this service myself over the years and I encouraged both my son and my husband to do so. It really helped them. And by doing so, it really helped *me*. I knew they had someone to talk to and I knew they could not talk to me at that point.

Being so incredibly *dependent* was very difficult for me on lots of levels. Poor Tommy was now in charge of absolutely *everything*, including the house. We are a team, and I couldn't show up for the game. I felt weirdly ashamed.

Being a caretaker is very hard and in some cases it can be sheer hell ….

I hear a strange sound. I turn and discover Terminal standing over my shoulder rubbing his hands with glee. "What, pray tell, do you want NOW?"
"Is this the part where you talk about what a control freak you can be? I LOVE it! Tommy is such a nice guy…."
"Do they make a special duct tape that works on you? I told you to leave me alone for a while."
"I did! Now I'm back!"
"Well, aren't I the lucky duck? GET OUT!" I grab my stapler and wave it menacingly at him.

Unphased, he says, "When are you going to be done then? I'm bored."

"What are you? Five? I'll be done when I am done. Why don't you go clean your room or something?"

"You sound exactly like your mother. Besides, MY room is already clean."

"Well, go clean MY room then. Frankly, I don't care what you do – just as long as you do it SOMEWHERE ELSE!"

"Promise me that you are going to discuss your control issues first."

"Fine. I was just getting to that. Just go. Now. Go NOW. Bye-bye. See ya'." He left.

And we are on to my control issues, I guess! I am a bit reticent, I will admit, but….

Back to the house. In the beginning it seemed to be OK. Tommy would clean things and I would lay on the couch and volunteer information and instructions on how to do it "right". This didn't go over so well for some odd reason. I realized I was being a control freak about the whole matter, but I couldn't seem to *recognize* it while I was actually *doing* it and therefore *stop* doing it.

Critique the man who is your lifeline! Now there's a brilliant plan! I'm *such* a superstar!

" 'Superstar' would not be my word for it…" I hear from the other room. I forget that he is in my mind.
"But then again, YOU aren't writing it now are you?"

I don't think there is a married couple out there that doesn't have go-rounds over housework. My husband has always pulled his own weight in that department (to a degree anyway), but he has also carried the archaic notion that by virtue of my sex the responsibility is ultimately *mine*. He cooks, I clean the kitchen – I get that. I cook, I clean the kitchen. Never quite sure how that one worked. Basically, this boils down to "I clean the kitchen". You get the idea.

Now he's upset: "I'm doing all the housework. I clean the kitchen at least twice a day (*true story*) and you don't appreciate it. All you do is criticize me." (*Also a true story.*)

Terminal was right; I had become my mother. Damnit! I'm NIT PICKING!!!! Having been on the receiving end of that delightful trait, I immediately apologized and promised myself and him that I would shut the hell up. Who cares if he doesn't get with the details? It's his problem to figure it out. They are his details now, not mine. My plan was to retire my mouth *now*.

Or not.

Control Brain puts on a new outfit and takes over again. I try a new approach: "Honey? I'm not trying to criticize you. *Really*, I am not. But I know how you like things to be and I can see that, despite your efforts, they aren't getting there. I'm just trying to teach you a couple *little bitty things* that might make this easier. That's all. I'm sorry."

"Congratulations! You successfully retired your mouth for 42 seconds. I'm so proud."
"What?" I ask, affecting my most innocent tone.
"Again! You sound just like your mother when you were caretaking her! Might I remind you that you found it annoying as hell when she did this to you? Not to mention EXTREMELY transparent. Do you really think Tommy can't see through this pathetic and CONTROLLING act of yours right now?"
"He doesn't seem upset to me!"
Have you ever seen a figment of your imagination roll his eyes at you? Lemme tell you, it is something to behold. "Do you remember your mother and her arbitrary butter fixation?"

I had to think about that one. My mother had died about a year before I had been diagnosed and I had been her caregiver. It was really hard at first. And yes, I remembered the God-forsaken butter fights. She wanted *unsalted* butter and when I got that she would throw a complete fit and tell me that she told me before she wanted *salted* butter. When I bought her salted butter we did it again in reverse until I finally was so loaded up on butter in my refrigerator that it was paramount to insanity. Then, once she found options were readily available, she adopted a *new* approach, just like I had done, and I wound up making two slices of toast, one with sweet butter and one with salted butter. She was making me batshit crazy and, while I definitely wanted to take good care of her, I also wanted to strangle her.

"Is that what I am doing here?"
"You tell me. He brings you a bowl of oatmeal and you announce that you don't like it because he didn't put a pinch of salt in it. Where would you have gone with that if your mother had done that to you? And don't tell me you would be interested in the culinary advantages of that, or whatever fancy bullshit you may conjure up to disguise your frustration. You would have verbally let loose on your mother. I know it; you know it!"
"You don't understand, we critique each other's food all the time."
"DO you? Maybe it's more like YOU critique HIS food all the time. You have to stop this." He pauses and says in a much gentler tone, *"You had a little dish of salt right in front of you. Might I remind you that he was the one who thought to put it there? He truly loves you, Sharon."*

He's right. What am I *doing*? I'm very sick, I'm very incapable and *what*? Now I'm a *dictator*? I finally stopped. Right then. Right there.

It is so easy to be critical of your caregiver. Sooooo easy. We forget that they aren't us. They are trying to stand in our stead, but that doesn't make them *us!* Being a caretaker is no picnic with some crazy control freak trying to play supervisor. You don't need a mean caregiver, that's for sure, but I betcha it is people like me that make 'em mean.

The truth of the matter is that it is harder to *receive* care than to *give* it, for me at least. It's really not about things being done "my way", but more because I can no longer do them myself and doubt I ever will be able to do them again. Those silly things are the things I have to let go of; symbolic of what I *really* have to let go of; like my *life*. I guess I'm practicing. But I have to try that without it being at someone else's expense.

4. CHEMO CLASS

I'm in a wheelchair full time now. I'm wearing some sort of horrific back brace that barely fits me due to my stomach extraordinaire which seems to keep filling up by the hour no matter how many times I get the damn thing drained. (The first time they took 5.2 liters out and *that wasn't even all of it*). I am the QUEEN of pillows – everywhere I try to sit requires at least five. And I *hurt*. I hurt like there is no tomorrow. I can barely swallow, I can only take a sip of water at a time, although all I want to do is chug a huge glass – to the point where I cry when I see one of my dogs just lapping it up out of their bowl. I can't burp but I feel like I have to. I ate about five Tums once and was able to burp one small burp and take one whole swallow of water. It was manna from Heaven, I swear it was. Then I threw it up. I can't fart, if I pee it hurts (not like a UTI, just a horrific pain of letting it out) and then it is only a tiny amount. I learned that "big girl panties" are diapers at this juncture in my life. If I could physically swallow enough to actually *eat*, it came right back up. (Funny how in one direction my body totally rebelled, but no problem in the reverse).

At night, if I could swallow them, my pain meds would knock me out enough to sleep. Tommy would wake up several times a night just to check to see if I was still breathing.

I was actively dying and we both knew it.

When they first told me two to four months left, I could *kind of* see it. But six weeks after that, I *believed* it. I was tied to a train track and that train was coming right on schedule. There was only one slim hope for me and that was chemo. But it was taking a long time to get going.

The first thing we had to do was to go to "Chemo Class". I kid you not – that is what it was called. I had visions of sitting in a room with a bunch of other "newbies" taking turns writing "wig" and "nausea" on the chalkboard to see if we could graduate to the next level – the actual chemo; my last bastion of hope.

Turns out that wasn't far from the truth. Let me preface this by saying that I don't have a lot of tolerance for this kind of thing. While there was no chalkboard and it was just Tommy and I, this was still complete *hell*.

The first thing we had to do was go sit in a little room and watch a 20-minute video on chemotherapy and what to expect. Eighteen minutes of this was dedicated to losing one's hair and how to fit a wig. I kid you not. People are spending thousands of dollars flying to obscure countries to hike up mountains and have some medicine man throw snake oil and god-only-knows what else on them to avoid putting this stuff in their bodies and we are supposed to be worried about if my new *wig* is going to fit? *Brilliant*.

But that was the *good* part. Step two was something beyond description – but I am going to try, nonetheless.

We get into a room with a nurse. It takes about 40 seconds for us to realize that she is extremely disorganized and unprepared. Three minutes into it, I'm very clear on the part where she has absolutely zero sense of humor. None. Zero. Zip. Humor and sarcasm being my survival reflex action, this was hard for me. I was trapped like a rat in a room with the single most naïve, insecure woman I had encountered in a long, long time.

About an hour in, I am starting to lose my patience. And apparently it is becoming rather obvious. I noticed Terminal is here. Asleep. Sitting on the floor next to me. I kicked him.

"What was THAT for?"
"Wake up, asshole. If I have to suffer, so do you!"
"Hey! You are here trying to draft my eviction notice – why should I participate in that?"
"Don't act like you have nowhere else to go." I felt like I was sending my teenager to go couch-surf for awhile, lest I strangle him.
"Because I don't have anywhere else to go. I'm stuck in the middle with you, babe."
And then he breaks into the Stealers Wheel song, "Clowns to the left of me, jokers to the right, here I am, stuck in the middle with you..."
"Shut up. Just shut up already."

Somehow she notices my annoyance. Did I say that last out loud?

"Sharon? I get the distinct feeling you are angry and you don't want to do this!"

"I'm in excruciating pain. No, I don't want to sit here and listen to this much longer."

Mind you, we are about an hour in.

The pain comment is dismissed in a snap, "Well, this is very *important* stuff. It won't be much longer. I need you to pay attention." Terminal was now sticking his tongue out at her, *but I needed a rifle.*

On and on she drones. I can't eat any raw fruits or vegetables or raw meat or fish if I am "that" sort of person (which I am) due to contaminants. No hot tub for the same reason and we have to keep the animals from drinking out of the toilets for a few days after chemo. I'm none too happy about any of this, but *whatever*. I can't eat anyway. I'm trying like hell to keep my face reasonably pleasant but I know my smile was as fake as that sports guy on Shark Tank.

Rage was coming. Tommy kept patting my hand and giving me the "just hang in there look" punctuated with the worried look. He told me later that it was like watching a volcano getting ready to blow.

She had a bunch of papers in her hands that she kept rifling through, talking to herself, saying nothing of consequence for another half hour and finally I had had *enough*.

Enough. Enough. Enough. And the volcano erupted.

"I'm leaving."

"No! It will only be a little bit longer! I have to explain this to you *thoroughly*!" I seriously considered telling her that she was failing at that miserably, but stopped myself when Terminal pointed out that she just might decide to start all over again.

"Those papers in your hand – are they for us to take?"

"Yes."

"Do they have bullet points on them?"

"Yes!"

"News flash! *I can read.* And I am *done*. Not another minute. Finish up with him." Yes, I threw my husband straight under the bus and went and laid down in the car. The pain was off the hook and *one* of us was going to die. Me or her. My money was on *her*.

God love him, I don't know how he managed to hold all that together for however much longer it took, but two hours and twenty minutes was much more than enough for me.

Finally, he got in the car. "You OK?"

"Just get me home. I'm sorry for throwing you under the bus like that."

"Not a problem. I kept telling you to calm down, but I could see it was not going to happen."

"Dear GOD! That was INSANE! Is she going to be my *nurse*? I mean, she seems nice enough, but I ...oh dear God... OK... whatever I have to do, I will do."

"It will be OK honey. We will make it work."

The Golden Word: "We".

I thought I was supposed to start chemo the next day or two. But they didn't call me. I had gotten my heart checked out and all the other requisite stuff I was supposed to do, so I was confused. I called. (Please remember that days are now *years* off my life. I am flat out of time.)

"Oh! You WANT to do the chemo? We were told you didn't want to do it!"

Dollars to donuts I bet I know what happened there. If I have learned anything at all by this point, I have learned that insecurities are downright dangerous. Not only to you, but also to others. Doubtless the nurse interpreted my refusal to go any farther with the class as a rejection of treatment. I should have been more specific; something like, "You sound like Charlie Brown's teacher and you are making me clinically insane."

"Then why, pray tell, would I have suffered myself through all of this crap, particularly 'Chemo Class'?"

I was able to start the next week. Mercifully, this poor woman was a traveling nurse and was leaving quite soon. When I went up for my preliminary blood tests, I heard her in the nurses' area and I could tell she was really very insecure and probably lonely. My heart softened then. I was just in a bad state and clearly lacking my normal humanity. Pain will do that to you, but it's no excuse. Well, *maybe*. Insecurities lead to membership in the All-About-Me-Gang. I had had enough of THAT lately. Damn near killed me.

"I think you have had enough of that for five lifetimes, if you want my humble opinion."
"And what, exactly, do you know about being humble?"

He has a toothy grin.

As I essentially learned *nothing* in my chemo class, I did learn a few things along the way. While chemotherapy is different for everyone, here are some things you can pretty much count on. (In no particular order)

1. Say good-bye to your taste buds. This doesn't last, but it's pretty obnoxious. There are four basic food groups of chemo. They are: metal, chalk, cardboard, or sawdust. (Not that I have ever actually *eaten* any of those things in my life, but that is what I *assume* they taste like). Then things that you once hated will suddenly show up on the scene and you will find them to be the most wonderful things in the whole world. Seriously, it's weird. For instance, I am not a sweet eater. I would have the obligatory bite of some dessert here and there, but wasn't much for it. But *now*? I'm blowing through fruit like it is going out of style. Chocolate? Ice cream? Look out baby! Vegetables, which I once loved, fell largely into the cardboard arena, except my least favorite, zucchini, which I am here to proclaim as the Food of the Gods. It's super weird.
    Forget processed foods. Some of my secret sins are a raw hot dog and baloney. I'm also a fan of those little processed cheese slices. OMG! ALL I could taste was the "processed" part of these things. It was as if my body was saying, "Duh!"
    Stay far away from pepper and just forget about wine. That tasted like someone had poured rubbing alcohol over black pepper and lemons. (Maybe I need to buy better wine?) But be patient, no matter how it goes for you. It passes and it's more important than you think. You *have* to eat. Protein

powder probably helped to save my life. Make a shake and just get it in you, even if it takes all day and it does taste like chalk.

2. Nausea. We all hear about this. Lots of puking. I was seriously concerned about this one. They give you anti-nausea medication. If it isn't working, talk to your doc right away – they can give you a second one that you can take in intervals. They work, but the trick is to stay up on them; stay ahead of the nausea, don't wait until you are wanting to throw up. I only had to take it the first week after each treatment.

3. Dry mouth. Redefined. Sudden and severe. You may think you have had this before. No, you have *not* – not like *this*. Lemon drops. Any sour candy. This is not cotton-mouth from smoking too much pot, people, this is in a class by itself. For me, it had a cute little way of showing up the second I had to swallow a pill.

4. Speaking of pills, potassium is a big player in this war and I gather that chemo likes to destroy it when you need it most. So they may give you a potassium pill among other things. Welcome to Pill Hell. If you think those giant calcium pills are hard to swallow, just wait until you give these bad boys a go. The good news is that they have no taste. The bad news is that they will dissolve the second you put them in your mouth and you will wind up with a mouthful of potassium *sand* which is nearly impossible to get down. Even with water. Dry mouth might come in handy here, but I never found that I could summon that on demand. Put it in yogurt, a little dish of soup – something. Or else you can just spit little particles of sand for the rest of the day.

5. Weird shooting and random pains. Remind yourself that this is the chemo attacking the cancer, which thinks it owns the place. You have the unfortunate role of hosting this party of bad guests. Just hang in there. It gets better.

6. The Nest. Prepare your world prior to chemo. I splurged and bought a new pillow and comforter for my couch. Never regretted a dime of it. It is my daytime nest. I'm cozy, I have all my shit there, I can eat there and I have the TV there. Prep your nest. TV trays are a good idea.

7. Take your temperature a lot. They will explain the importance of the white blood cell count to you; pay close attention. This is life or death time for you. Chemo will LEVEL your WBCC straight out the gate. Ideally you will get a booster shot to make more, but if they fall down on you, your worst case scenario is dying from the common cold and your best case scenario is a stint in the hospital and a good possibility that you will not be able to continue your chemo. DO NOT FUCK AROUND WITH THIS. Anything over 100.4 is hospital time. Call your doctor *immediately*. If you can't reach him/her – go to the ER. It will feel like 104.0, trust me.

8. Neuropathy. Once again, I knew nothing about this at all going in. It was due to a friend who has traversed this road herself and contacted me about some herbal supplement that she is using for neuropathy. I had no idea what she was talking about, but I said, "sure." Then I learned what this is. Yep, another chemo game!
    What happens with this one is that your feet and hands go numb, get all tingly, and, in my case, ice cold! This can extend itself, apparently, to becoming a lifetime issue, that can pretty much cripple you. Thankfully, it did not in my case.

Now, while "numb" may sound easy enough, fair warning: it moves its way into some sort of bizarre throbbing pain and can *really* hurt. And the aforementioned feet may fail you. I remember trying to get up once and screaming in pain. Mercifully, Tommy was there and caught me before I fell. Massage seems to be the obvious answer, but it wasn't for me. Getting the circulation going is a plus, but when he massaged my actual foot, it only rushed in the pain. Having him "pet" my feet and legs worked, however. Somehow, I could just focus on that. But when the pain really started to rock and roll, I used ice packs. Didn't take long, maybe five to ten minutes, but that seemed to calm everything down enough to go to sleep.

This can hit you in the knees and hips as well, as time goes on. And it's *sudden*. When it does, you will know. Suddenly you won't be able to take a step in any direction without the distinct possibility of going down. It's OK to use a walker. This too will pass. *Falling is not your friend.*

9. Constipation. I think this is inevitable and it is *hell*. Right after my chemo it was *baaaad*. I've learned, and suggest you do as well, to take stool softeners *prior* to treatment and continue for a few days. For me, this was the worst of it. The pain is remarkable and the process of "elimination" has taken up to four miserable hours. This is going to sound insane unless you wind up in my shoes – but try pooping standing up when the urge really hits. It *works*.

10. The Port. This is a thingy that is medically inserted in your chest. It has a tube that inserts into one of your veins and a round plastic area, with three bumps on it that is inserted just under your skin. The idea behind this gizmo is that it makes giving you an IV, or taking your blood much easier and a hell of a lot less painful. As a matter of fact, it can turn out to be a godsend. But what you need to know is that it is quick, easy and a REALLY good idea

5. CHEMO NUMBER ONE

This is scary. I don't want to go. But by the same token, I don't want to keep dying and living in the agony I am in. So off I go.

To be honest, and in retrospect, I think I was more nervous about spending hours upon hours hooked up to an IV, trapped like a rat, and sitting in a recliner (albeit a very comfortable one – but sitting was agony for me then, so who knew how it was going to go?)

Seven hours. SEVEN, they said. I don't think I've sat still for seven consecutive hours in my *life*! What if it hurts? What if I panic? What if, what if, what if????!!!!!!

Tommy was supportive in the extreme, but then, he wasn't privy to all the paranoia going on in my mind, either. He *was,* however, privy to the action I was taking to assuage the paranoia going on in my mind. If I needed to distract myself for seven hours, *dammit,* I was going to be *prepared.*

Here is what I brought:

My down comforter in case I got cold.

3 pillows because they are my life line.
My watercolor pens, pencils, paper and varying sundries
A book (hardback).
A change of clothes
A book on disk and a CD player with headphones (still haven't figured out how to do this stuff with my phone.)
And more food and beverages than I had consumed in the last 3 weeks, collectively.

I was good to go for a *month*.

Tommy carried it all out to the car without remark, got me in, arranged the requisite pillows around me and we began the one-hour journey into what I was *sure* was going to be *absolute hell*.

While Tommy made no comment in regards to all this, Terminal had PLENTY of comments, but managed to keep it down to a minimum.

"So! You are moving IN to the infusion room, I see!"
"I'm just being prepared."
"For what, exactly? Armageddon?"
"Chemo makes you sick. I'm already sick. And now I'm going to be MORE sick."
"Well, better pull that barf bag out of your glove box then, because I hear it also makes you puke."

With that, he, mercifully, shut up. I will say that I did *not* pull the barf bag out of my glove box. (I already had one packed.)

I went into the doctor's office and then was taken into the "Infusion Room" where several other people were there, seated in a circle. We were greeted by the nurses and everybody watched as Tommy brought in load after load of my stuff, culminating in a big puffy comforter.

After Tommy got me settled in the chair and left, someone asked me if it was my first treatment. I looked around the room. A couple of books, a cell phone or two with headsets…..

"Yeah," I responded with half my life surrounding my chair, "Is it *that* obvious?"

"You will be OK." A knowing smile and a return to their own business. But the empathy was clear.

"I told you so!"
"Oh goody. Look who's here! How fucking special."
"Where did you expect me to be? I go with you everywhere now. Just think of me as your own personal guide dog."
"OK, Spot, what would you know about chemo treatments?" It was a stupid question, and I knew it as soon as I said it, but what I *DIDN'T* know was that it would be the first of a long list of stupid questions I would ask over the next few months.
"I hate to break this to you, much as I love you, but you are not my first."

I grabbed my sketch pad. I decided to sketch his dumb ass. I didn't get much on the paper, but I got something bigger than a mere rendition of him.

I put his name on the top in big block letters "TERMINAL" and then it hit me like a ton of bricks. That was a game changer for me.

I *stared* at the word. I don't know why, but I had drawn squares underneath it – like big TV screens… and BAM! A terminal is a bus, rail, airplane station. *Think* about it – it's where you change destinations. You either go get in the car and go home, or you do a layover, then get on another bus and go to the next destination.

I closed my eyes and looked. I didn't see the bus marked "DEATH" in the terminal. At least not *yet*. And I realized that, against all apparent odds, I still had a choice of which bus I was going to get on. None of the destinations were clear to me yet, but at least I didn't see a big black bus looming about.

My perspective changed at that very moment.

I was no longer trying to get used to the idea of dying in a couple of months, I was fighting for my life *right* now. And I was going to get on a different bus, dammit.

At this point I was snapped out of my reverie by someone asking me about my art stuff. It's been a very long time since I have sketched or painted in public (decades actually) and I had forgotten that this absolutely fascinates people. For those of us who do it, we just *do* it – we don't think about it being a big thing, but for others it is pretty cool. Like when I see someone playing the piano – I'm mesmerized no matter how badly they do – it's so far away from myself and what I can do. What a thing to have that kind of talent!

"I can play the piano badly, if that is what you would like."
"No doubt you can. Let's just not and say you did."

I looked around the room then and everyone was *very* present. Someone asked me if I was the one who used to write the humor column in the local paper. That was years ago, so this surprised me. Amazingly enough, I finally stopped being embarrassed about bringing half the planet with me and being so damn pathetic. I was in a room full of people who were on the same path, who *understood*, who cared as much as they could in their own circumstances and who quietly and peacefully took me in with an acceptance that is rare in my life. I was scared, sick, weak, and, well... pretty much helpless. But, apparently *here*, that didn't render me useless. I was *not* null and void. I AM NOT NULL AND VOID! For the first time since my diagnosis, I wasn't defined by my cancer. I *mattered*.

The rest of the day proved enjoyable, actually. There is an unwritten code of understanding in that room. Everybody's chair is their personal bubble. You can sleep: everyone gets that and is respectful; you can read, everyone gets that also and is respectful; you can chat; or you can just simply BE!

Then there are the bags they hook you up to. If you are going in for the first time because you are pretty much on your last legs with metastatic cancer, this means *lots* of bags. I didn't get that memo. I thought it was one bag – the chemo, and then I was out of there.

But nooooo. More like six. It's just a series of things that they give you before and after the "big bags" which are chemo and in my case an immunosuppressant. Some of these bags are anti-nausea juice, Benadryl (sleepy time) and STEROIDS (zippy time)! The first treatment requires a lot of the last three to see how you handle the Big Two.

I didn't know any of this right then. I know they *told* me, but I was such a mess, that all I absorbed was that there were a hell of a lot of bags and some of them were *very* slow.

Finally, it was time to go home. Tommy came to get me and asked me how it went. I was as surprised as he was to hear me say it was OK. And I was *perky*. None of those things that I heard about chemo happened. I didn't get sick at all. Actually, I felt better than I had in weeks, months even. Then I had him take me out for a fast food burger and a strawberry shake. This – btw, is *beyond* out-of-character. But I could EAT! I chatted him up all the way home and kept it up until waaay late. At one point he pawned me off on our roommate.

I felt pretty good the next day too. Hey! This chemo stuff is GREAT! I'm Superwoman! I'm going to cruise *right* through this! I got this one, baby! Look out.

Welcome to Steroids. It's kind of like cocaine for the terminally ill. But, also like cocaine, what goes up, must come *down*.

And *look out*! Right down, baby, right down on the couch and unable to talk, much less move.

I don't remember much from the first week. All I remember is feeling all the sharp stabs and sudden shooting pains. This was different from (and on top of) the pain I was already in. The only comfort I had was in pain pills and telling myself that the pain was the chemo meeting the cancer and that it *had* to be a good thing.

My family said I looked like imminent death. I guess I looked like I *felt*.

It was in the second week that it got really interesting. I thought I was doing better, which I was, insomuch as I now could sit up, had adjusted to the taste of metal and friends, and was able to communicate in something more than a mumble. I also had the nausea pills dialed in and wasn't on the verge of throwing up every few minutes. I appreciated that. The pain had diminished a bit, and well, I was still *alive*. That had to count for something.

One of the big things with chemo is that it likes to use all the gas in your tank. That gas would be your poor white blood cells who valiantly go forth in your honor to slay the dragon. I'm going to go out on a limb here and say that mine were pretty worn out, having tried and failed with the stupid cancer. Then the chemo rolled in, and, well, little white cells with little white "surrender" flags were seen everywhere.

These little dudes are a big deal and if they fall down and go "boom", *so do you.*

What happened to me next is very noteworthy.

I'm pretty much a zombie at this point, but we have to go up to have more of my blood drawn and see how the little fellas are doing. We get there, Tommy wheels me in, and the little fellas are found to be wandering sadly around the battlefield, barely able to walk. The doctor gives me a shot. They tell me I have to come back the next day for another one. Whatever. Home we go. Tomorrow is another day. Thank you, Scarlett O'Hara.

6. THE SHIT STORM

This is so humiliating that I have debated even putting it in here but, as my purpose is to tell you what *might* happen and help you navigate through your own slice of hell on your way to recovery, here I go:

I'm not a constipation girl. I'm not a throw up girl. I am a *diarrhea* girl. Look at me cross-eyed and I'm getting the runs. OK?

Welcome to chemo. Welcome to constipation. I had no clue this was coming "down the pike" (HA! I'm such a wit!). I was pretty much brain dead when I went to "chemo class" and if this information was given, I missed it.

Chemo constipates you. *Big time.*

I know I haven't pooped in a few days but I also know I haven't eaten in a few days to speak of. We were on our way to the doctor's office, which is an hour away. Tommy packs me and my eight million pillows in the car and off we go.

Then my bowels start moving. As this hasn't happened in a while,

40

I don't think much of it. We are only a few minutes up the road and suddenly my body means *business*. I tell him we need to stop. I have to "go".

He thinks I can hold it. I'm pretty sure he is *dead wrong*.

"OH my God, this is so humiliating. I don't think I can write this!"
"Yes you can. Besides, it's funny."
"FUNNY???"
"OK, not funny for YOU, but maybe funny for others. Make it funny." He fires me a cheesy little grin and ducks my swing. "Too soon?"

It's cold and drizzly outside. I live in the country, so it isn't like there is a gas station on every corner. But we are nearing a gated community where part of our family lives. (Meaning, we can get in).

We drive by their house and no one is there. I'm pretty desperate at this point, so we head to a park where we know there is a bathroom.

I'm holding on for all I'm worth and my husband's now driving as *slowly* as he possibly can. He will probably say this was to avoid bouncing me around, but it sure felt passive aggressive to me!

And then it is simply *too late*. Days upon days of body waste has just cut loose. Nothing I can do about it. The relief was overwhelming, but so was the horror of what was happening. Over and *over* again.

We pulled into this very public spot but the weather was on my side – nobody was there. *Thank God.*

It was absolutely horrifying. But you do what you have to do, right? This isn't about being brave. This is simply about immediate survival. Off go the pants and big girl panties. Lemme tell you – Depends are no match for this kind of deluge.

It's all down my legs. The only thing I can say about it is that it is

41

warm. Disgusting as hell, but *warm*.

Then it is on my shirt because of my hands and now I am naked and no longer warm. Tommy helps me into the glorified outhouse and we start trying to clean me up. Let me tell you that ice water and those cheap brown paper towels just don't cut it. But I did! I cut loose again all over the floor. Then *again* in the toilet. Literally, shit was *everywhere*. I was shaking like a leaf, while desperately trying to clean up. There was no way anything remotely close to "clean" was possible.

Tommy was heaving outside.

Not my sexiest moment. Nope. Nothing like standing naked in a public parking lot, half covered in your own feces and watching your spouse throw up to complete the picture of "Just Not So Sexy Anymore."

"Maybe you should write a song. I could sing it!"
"Seriously?"
"Well, you gotta admit it would be a catchy song title."

I had no time to respond to *that* as Tommy was hurrying me to the car. We headed back home and I called the nurse I was going to see. The same woman we had gone through chemo class with. She informed us that "it didn't matter" and that she could only wait 20 more minutes for me.

This timeline is a physical impossibility and regardless of her "come as you are" attitude I was *pretty sure* she had no idea what she was saying and I was damn sure I wasn't driving an hour naked except for a mysterious brown sheen all over my legs. I negotiated an extra ten minutes and we flew home. Let's face it, I may have *looked* tan, but I sure as hell didn't smell like coconut oil.

"I'm too sexy for my car, too sexy for my car. Too sexy by far" is now playing as my uninvited background music.

42

Oh joy. He keeps doing his best "model" walk and having entirely too much fun at my expense. *Again.*

"Just stop. Please."
"Do you know who sings that?"
"No, Terminal, and right at this juncture I care less than I know!"
"'Right Said Fred'. That's the name of the band. I love it!"

While I could stand on my own, walking was not an option and neither was going up the eight stairs to my house in any sort of a timely manner. We had to hurry. *Really* hurry.

I was pretty fucking sick and I knew it. So, I would do anything, ANYTHING to make that appointment. (This was the day I wound up in the hospital). But what "anything" entailed was becoming quite extreme.

Tommy got me in our courtyard which is the closest spot to my car, handed me the hose and ran up the stairs to gather the dishwashing soap, a towel, sweatpants and a T-shirt. Meanwhile I took a shower of ice water in my courtyard. Did I mention it is about 40 degrees outside? Back in the car we go. We actually made it. I could not believe I had just done that. Funny thing, that nurse had no other appointments that day, but instead stuck around to watch the other nurses and my doctor scrambling to save my life. She's lucky I was so out of it.

"There. There it is in print. My most humiliating moment. Ta-da!"
"You could have been funnier. Besides, it's not your most embarrassing moment. Remember when you had to bring in a stool sample?"
"How in the world do you know about THAT?"
"You have a lot of files in here. A whole roomful, actually, right next to the Thrift Store."
"What?! And you feel free to just go rummaging about – is that it?"
"Yes. Consider it research. You are a writer and I am your research assistant. We are a TEAM! I wonder if you have anything that resembles a research assistant outfit?"

"Trust me on this: No."

He had a point. *That* was not my most embarrassing moment ever. I have told *that particular* story many times in my life and it *is* hilarious. It is funny in retrospect. I have no retrospect here.

"It's not funny."
"Yea, but you did enjoy the shower. I remember that!"
"I think the word 'enjoy' is a bit of a stretch, don't you? I suspect that anyone who has recently been dipped in feces would 'enjoy' washing it off. That hardly makes the whole freezing event 'ENJOYABLE!'"

I have to admit, despite the cold of it (I quickly went numb anyway), I *do* remember the light of the day. The light was so perfect. This is the visual artist in me speaking and I don't know how to describe it. So clear, muted, but clear.

"You said it was almost white. A white light."
"That better not be THE white light – the one people talk about seeing when they die and come back? Tell me it wasn't, Terminal!"
He shrugged, *"I dunno...maybe. You were pretty close right then."*
"Don't remind me."
"And you thought about that shower all the way up to the doctors. So you must have enjoyed it On some level."
"I thought about the possibility of putting in an outdoor shower there. THAT is what I thought about."
"See? You enjoy that kind of thing!"
"Let me clarify this for you; I thought about putting in a HOT shower!"

From that day forward we started carrying a go-bag with us everywhere we went. In it is a change of clothes, extra Depends, soap, rags, etc. We also carry a couple gallons of water. I strongly recommend this precautionary move. And for the ladies, pack some baby wipes. You have to keep the feces out of your whoo-who. The last thing you need right now is a UTI.

7. THE HOSPITAL

We go to see my doctor the next day and things are not pretty. Not *remotely* pretty. I feel lousy, and apparently, I am now running a fever and some of the little white cell dudes are now seen falling flat on their faces in the middle of the battlefield. I don't know *what* is going on. But my medical team sure as hell does and I can hear them, one by one, trading off the phone until it finally wound up being my actual doctor yelling at some guy from my insurance company.

My insurance has denied the shot I desperately needed despite being told that I could die without it.

I don't think I fully understood this at that time, but they sure as hell did. They were *royally* pissed off and visually upset. I heard what they said, but kept thinking that if I could just go home and sleep.... I now know I would not have woken up. Powerless to argue the point, I sat there while my doctor told me a story about some other patient and told us we needed to go DIRECTLY to the closest ER and he would call ahead. Without this shot, I was going to die, and very soon. Maybe in mere hours.

I understand this now. But at that moment, I really could not completely grasp it. I just remember my doctor explaining to me how imperative it was that I do *not* go home and play my favored "ignore it and it will go away" game. I had to go *directly* to the hospital. The phone call had resonated with me, certainly, as did their insistence. But I didn't fully absorb the *magnitude*. I guess it was simply par for the course, in my mind. I was dying. That was not new information to me. Pretty much from the minute I was diagnosed, I had put my head down and simply plowed ahead with blinders on. I just gotta do what I gotta do. That was my mantra. Tell me what to do and I will do it.

Honestly, I think I just had enough. I had simply had *enough*. I couldn't take my emotional response any further than that. I was tapped out. Tommy got it, though.

So away we went. None of my medical team wanted me to go to the hospital that was literally right across the street, but they decided that it was imperative that I do so due to the expediency of the thing.

Oh. My. God. What a fiasco. What a bloody fiasco. First off, the place is under construction. This is not an issue except for me, *the one who shall stay away from all germs*, and is now forced to use the blue room outside. Wheelchair accessible or *not*, an outhouse is probably *not* the best idea. After dousing myself with hand sanitizer (that stuff weirds me out – where does it go? Am I absorbing Clorox into my body? Sounds like *another* genius plan – you wait people, Hand Sanitizer Cancer is coming, just give it a decade).

After that we go into the building and meet the Covid Cop. Yes, this is the guy who always wanted to make the police force, but didn't pass the psychological part of the test thus failed because *he should never have a gun*. He's security for the hospital instead, and he is going to *catch* those evil covid people who are trying to LIE to him and say they don't have covid but ONE LOOK at them proves that they are *highly suspect*.

Officer Idiot, as it turns out, has a partner in crime at the desk. This would be the single most nasty woman I have ever encountered in a hospital setting. Not to mention the single *loudest* person I have ever encountered in a hospital setting. Tommy explains to her that our doctor called ahead and I am to go right in, but Miss Angry at the World tells him he has to leave right now because nobody except patients are to be in the area. Tommy leaves. The female creature tells me to go to the end of the hall and wait there. I can't.

"I told you to move along. We have other people waiting!" (No, I am not exaggerating)

"I *can't*. I need *help*." My wheelchair is a transport wheelchair I got from a friend. What this means is that it doesn't have the big wheels so you can push it yourself, just four small wheels. If I could stand up and push the damn thing, why would I be *in* it?

Begrudgingly, she pushes me down the hall and parks me at the end of some random corridor; assuring me that someone will be with me shortly, and splits.

The place is *freezing*. This is due to the freezing weather outside and the fact that the first hall has no finished walls; some flapping plastic, but definitely no insulation.

I don't have my phone. Fucking *fabulous*. I'm going to die in a hallway. I'm shivering and I'm incapable of getting any help.

"Look around. Interest yourself" It's Terminal. Oh Joy.
"What?"
"Engage. Check out your surroundings". I look; there are three other guys in this 30-foot hallway. One is asleep, the other two are hanging their heads so low they might have been dead.
"Why? What do you care, anyway? You should be happy as hell. Isn't your whole goal to see me dead?" (I realize that that is a self-pitying and largely pathetic statement. But as I was, in that moment BOTH self-pitying AND pathetic, it seemed honest, if nothing else.)
"No, actually. My goal is to test you with your own mortality to see what you ultimately choose to do. You are a people person. How

many times has THAT skill saved your life?"

I said nothing.

How many times indeed? I could write a whole book on that one. People have been my life's work. I hadn't thought about that.

I will try. Unfortunately, the three of my corridor comrades appear to be barely living corpses and clearly not available for comment. One got collected and another one just finally got up and left. I didn't blame him. But not to worry! A new one came and joined us, sent along by Miss Angry at the World. He was very chatty. Apparently, mom dropped him off *again* on a 5150 (mental). Oh, goody. Now it is me, the guy I'm afraid has *actually* died, and Spin Bunny (rehab, Mom, the kid needs *rehab*). I was trying to scoot my way just enough to see around the corner.

5150 was *all over it*. He was appalled that I was sitting there for so long, offered me his coat, and we swapped stories the best I could. He was mad about my situation and pushed me a little farther down the hall toward Miss Angry at the World. Just a few feet down the hall. Still 30 feet away from any other human being. He was lovely and he was truly a gentleman.

Then I get spotted by her and Officer Covid. By the grace of all things holy, Tommy had come back in and heard her admonishing me to get back around the corner. It had been almost an hour.

Despite their protests, Tommy came to me and asked if anyone had come to see me yet. I said, "No. Get me the *hell* out of here; I am NOT dying in this God-forsaken hallway."

Miss Angry at the World was *beside* herself, spitting and hissing like a feral cat. Not *only* had Tommy broken protocol, now he was trying to *steal* me. He told her that we didn't have any more time to wait. She fired off with: "What do you want me to do? Kick a patient out of their bed because *she* is so important?" *Noooo*, but we *do* expect to be told if the hospital is full (it wasn't) and we must wait for a bed. Was I supposed to sit in the hallway with Mr.

5150 for two days while we waited for someone to go home? Those were *my* thoughts. My husband was another story altogether. Mercifully, he had the sense to get us out of there before the Covid Cop grabbed his golden opportunity and Tommy wound up in Hospital Security Jail and I wound up back in the Hallway of Hell.

Off we went to the next hospital, a half hour or more away. I called my Doctor to tell him what we were doing and to call ahead. All he said was "Hurry.

That hospital was a whole different ball game. They were actually *waiting* for me and I was whisked away immediately. For five days I was poked and on an IV. I had my temperature taken at every turn and it would *not* break. I was in a little room by myself and not allowed to leave it. The Nurses had to wear paper over-gowns to even come near me. *One more germ and I was done for.*

I was never going home. I was going to die there. I was sure of it. I slept round the clock for three days (as much as one can in a hospital). I called Tommy once a day. It was all I could do. I was really, really fucked up. And I was *terrified.* But Terminal was right on with the people thing. Those nurses were little angels flitting about in my world. They kept me going, listened to me, dried my tears, helped me sit up, brought me warm blankets ALL the time, disconnected my room phone after I threatened to throw it out the window because the damn cafeteria kept calling me and were trying to poison me and I decided I hated them very much. (Except the ones that brought me said food. They were nice.)

Finally, my fever broke and *stayed* that way. They never did figure out what sort of virus I had, but they did figure out a combination of antibiotics that worked. Good enough for me! I lived and I was going *home.*

When Tommy came to get me, it was a *beautiful* day. It had rained the entire time I was there. Everything was full of color and just vivid. We took the long way home, just going slowly. I was so happy and relieved to be with my husband and safe and alive and going home.

After that and a long nap, I realized that I felt better. Not just pre-hospital-sick better, but better-better. I was still in pain, but much less so.

That was the first time I *knew* that the chemo was working. I hoped like hell this was not something I would be doing every three weeks, but if it was – *so be it. The chemo was working.*

8. CHEMO NUMBER TWO

This time I did not bring the *whole* farm with me. Only half of it. Everybody was happy to see me and remarked on me having some color back. Apparently, I was white as a sheet on their last sighting. I didn't know because I had given up on the mirror quite a long time ago. If I did look in the mirror it was to make sure I was still breathing. But I felt better and was encouraged that this showed.

Onto the scale I went and I had lost 12 pounds! I definitely had that to lose and must admit it was nice to see the 150's again. (158). While it's one hell of a way to go about losing weight, I was happy to see it. Not only for the obvious reasons, but because it was further proof that the chemo was working. My belly was *shrinking*. I had visual *proof.*

Tommy was given paperwork that the doctor had filled out so he could apply for family leave when his vacation and sick time ran out. I wanted to see it and he wanted to go. He had a golf date and the poor man needed a break from me, so no fault there, but *dammit*, I want to see the papers! I only got to look at the first page. "IS THE PATIENT TERMINAL?" The answer surprised me a little bit. I was expecting a simple "Yes" but it said, "Maybe. To be determined upon completion of treatment." I waved Tommy off for his day.

"Maybe." *Wow*. I am not stupid and I realize that treatment is out of my hands, but *still*… for the first time in a couple of months, I have a 'maybe'; a little *hope*. It was like being a drowning person and the only rope they can throw you is frayed and tattered, and yet one tiny tendril of the unraveled life I used to call my own managed to drop down into the water. You better believe I grabbed that thing and hung on for all I was worth.

I go get in my chair and they hook me up. My first bag goes fine, and a little way into bag number two, I'm chatting away and BAM! All of a sudden everything was yellow (don't ask me to explain this because I can't) and I felt *really* weird. I managed to call out to the nurse and say that something was wrong. Next thing I know I can't breathe, much less talk.

The whole ordeal only took a minute or two. Kerrylea, my nurse, remained very calm, unhooked my drip and Rosa, the second nurse, wheeled over the oxygen tank. I was able to breathe again pretty quickly and things stopped being yellow.

That is what went on outside of me, what went on in my *brain* was nowhere near that organized.

"OMG, I'm going to die. Right here, right now. This is it."
"Stop panicking. Don't try to breathe. You know that will only make things worse."
"OH SURE! Stop breathing. Gotcha. Grow a pair of lungs, asshole, I'm a HUMAN; breathing is a big part of what we do!!!!"
"You are not going to die today. Do you want to die today?"
"Would I be subjecting myself to all this if I wanted to die?"
"Considering the grand scheme of things in your life right now that you are handling with a fair amount of grace, you sure can make a fuss over the little shit." And with a smirk he wandered off.

I came back to the moment at hand to find all my comrades in chairs watching me expectantly with worried expressions on their faces (apparently I had been regaling everyone with some story when they turned yellow on me) and my nurse on her knees in front of me and the other one standing over me. I have to hand it to those two. They never let their panic show. That, right there, was a lifeline and a half.

"Well, THAT was fun!" I said, wide eyed.

Kerrylea smiled at me and said I had a reaction to the drug (which I assumed was the chemo) and she had unhooked me and was now giving me fluids. And not to worry, of course.

OK, situation handled! Then a few people in the room shared similar stories with me and I was fine to carry on. Until....

"OK, now we have to hook you back up. That is a very *important* bag and you have to have it."

Lemme tell you, I did NOT see that coming.

"Say WHAT???!! You *what?*"

She repeated herself.

"Wait a *minute*. Let's *review,*" I say as I put my hand up to stop her. "That stuff just tried to *kill* me, and your plan is to do it *again*? What? Five minutes on, five minutes being resuscitated, then back on, over and over? Color me *unusual*, but I'm not sure I'm *comfortable* with this plan!"

"Oh, we just need to slow it down. You handled it just fine last time so we tried to speed things up for you. If I slow it down, you will be just *fine.*"

I had visions of her going home and talking to her sweetie about work.
"How was your day, Dear?"

"Oh, the usual, a couple near-death experiences, but it was difficult to get one of them unglued from the ceiling......"

I begged for recess. I had to regroup.

"Terminal? You there?"
"Where else would I be?"
"Not so sure about this."
"Well, like I told you before. You have choices. You know what they are and it's up to you."

Then he wandered off to his room singing George Michael, 'You gotta have Faith.' (At least he could carry a tune. I don't know *what* I would have done if he couldn't.)

But he was right. I *had* to trust her. Trust has always been a challenge for me. I trust in pieces, I guess, but *completely*? With my *life*? It was true, also, that I had a choice in this matter. I could say no, and die, or trust her and maybe live. Woo-hoo! How is THAT for a choice?

So, after recess she hooked me back up. The whole room watched me like a hawk as I nervously prattled on about God-only-knows-what until I forgot all about it. (Those poor, patient people).

Giving it to me slowly meant extra hours on my time – three to be exact. The last couple hours were just me and Kerrylea. The office was long closed and dark, my doctor was ferreted away in his office and it was just us two getting to know each other. It was really a gift. No question this woman had just saved my life and I was thrilled to discover her sense of humor and other talents. I had found a *friend*. Terminal told me once that it was *people* that would save me. At the time he was referring to my love of people, but I was fast learning that it was also quite literal.

When Tommy showed up, I told him about what happened and he said in his annoyingly cavalier way, "Oh, so you had a reaction to the chemo, but it's all OK now?"

Kerrylea wasn't havin' it. "Not a 'reaction'. This wasn't a simple *reaction*; this was an *anaphylactic type* reaction and she could have *died*."

Whooo Baby! I guess there was no further chance of Tommy minimalizing THAT one! I have to admit that I loved her for that moment!

But I also saw, then, how scared *she* had been and admired even more how she had held that at bay for my sake. Not many people can do that.

On the way home I was smiling ear to ear, chatting about this and that (I love steroids) but inside, anaphylactic shock be *damned*; I had a balled-up thread of hope in my hand and I wasn't letting go. It was the word "Maybe."

9. THE FIRST HAIR EPISODE

Friday was my pre-chemo doctor visit where they take my blood to make sure I still have some and also my checkup. It went really well and I'm cleared for chemo number 3 (my halfway mark). I am doing well and I'm grateful for it - I can walk around now without playing "weebles wobble but they don't fall down," I can eat food without it tasting like good old metal, cardboard, sawdust and chalk. I'm not in pain to speak of anymore. Anyone who suffers from chronic pain will appreciate the value of *that*. My cancer was not caught quickly so by the time I got *into* chemo it had a pretty strong hold on me. Lemme tell you, that shit hurts. Mercifully, that pain is *gone*. All I have to do is contend with chemo's little bag of tricks. Trust me, I can lay on the couch and eat chalk and be nauseous for a week every few weeks. In the grand scheme of what I have been through since July*, that is nothing.*

When you first get going with chemo there is a big fixation on whether or not you are going to lose your hair. Seriously, it's the number one thing they tell you to expect (with my type of chemo, anyway). Having been on this path for a bit now, I assure you that there are *many* other things you should be aware of, but apparently the loss of the hair is a really big deal. I was duly informed by all the powers that be to expect this right away, no later than mid-session on Chemo number two.

Right after that comes another big wig talk - I could just think about it as a "chance to experiment with new looks and styles." That intrigued me for a minute, but when they didn't have a glittery Rod Stewart/ Tina Turner number, I pretty much moved on to the beanie. I don't go anywhere anyway.

Chemo number one does nothing to my hair. I thought it was going to *kill* me, but my hair went unscathed. About a week in, however, I had Brandon and Tommy shave my head. This was due to some very good advice passed along to me by an old friend. She said there are two ways to go about this - one, take control and just do it of my own volition or two, wake up a victim of the whole thing, yet again, in the middle of the night with my hair all over me and my pillow. I opted for plan A.

Almost to chemo number three, my hair is still intact (I even had eyebrows) and my shaved head is now covered in something strikingly akin to Velcro. It seems to be growing back mostly gray except for a long, skinny patch of brunette on the top. Insomuch as I can tell, I will be returning as some sort of reverse image of Cruella d'Vil.

Towards the end of my visit with my doctor, I removed my hat and he noticed my Velcro.

"I see your hair is starting to grow back. That's a good sign."

"I never lost it." He stares at me, clearly confused, so I clarify, "I shaved it. I am Woman, Hear Me Roar? That kinda deal."

"You haven't lost it from the chemo? Well, you might *not* then. Some women don't, but it's rare. Some lose just a little."

I just sat there looking at him for a moment.

"What's wrong?" He asks.

"I just don't know what to say to you right now, Doc."

There was no way in hell I could have figured out all those mixed emotions right then.

Seriously? Where does one go with *that?*

On the way home, I tried to sort it out in my mind. Of course, part of me wanted to strangle him for convincing me that losing my hair was an absolute and part of me wanted to shoot myself for jumping the gun. As I obsessively tugged on my eyebrows to see if they were remaining intact (I will admit to doing that ever since) I heard a sound coming from the back of my mind. I tried to ignore it, but I knew it was futile. It was Terminal and he was just *cracking up*. Clearly, he has a point to make, but in his typical fashion he is going to have some fun at my expense first.

"OK, Mr. Mirth. What the hell is so damn funny?"
"Oh nothing." This from the guy who is half doubled over in laughter.
"Nothing my eye. Out with it."
"What happened to the girl who took great pride in her lack of vanity, eh? I remember how CLEAR you were on the whole subject. Ironically taking great pride in your self-proclaimed lack of pride. Looks like the literal translation of 'I am woman, hear me roar' is 'I am a hypocrite watch me face plant'." Peels of laughter.
"Once again I want to punch you, Terminal. Like this isn't bad enough, I have to have the joker living in my head taunting me. Damn, you are mean!"
"I'm not mean. I am ACCURATE!"
"Laughing at someone else's expense is mean, Terminal."

OOOOOHHHH, a small moment for me. He HATES it when the tables get turned. He has a terrible reputation for being an asshole and I've learned that he is very sensitive about it. Not that he doesn't *deserve* it; riding into someone's parade and announcing that it is over mid-stream is not exactly how to win friends and influence people.

This is going to be a short-lived victory for me and I know it, but I'm enjoying it.

"OK. I'm sorry. I'll quit being mean if you quit checking your eyebrows every ten seconds." I immediately withdraw my hand from my face. "But you have to admit, Sharon, it is kind of funny."

Humor is the one place he and I seem to be able to meet in the middle, and while I know that the bigger subject of vanity must be explored (whether I like it or not), it *is* funny. Ironic.

At this point he heads to his projector and plays the "Great Head Shaving Episode of 2021" back to me.

I was determined. I really did not want some sudden hair episode (and to my understanding it is right then, right there, all at once, in huge handfuls). It seemed horrifying to me. What if I lose it in the grocery store or someplace public like that? Can you *imagine*? Go to hand the cashier your money with a big clump of hair on it? Yea, no. So I duly announce to my son and husband that we are doing this and we are doing it *now*.

The resistance was huge. I understood why, but I could not afford to look at it from their perspective. For them this was a huge reality check. I needed it to be simply part of the process, *done and over*. An experience we can remember forever. A bonding family moment. (Or whatever other wanna-be Hallmark lie I was attaching to it). Protests came in along with my husband's favored "I will do it tomorrow" routine, but I knew it was now or never for me and so I grabbed the scissors and just started hacking it off myself. Now that I looked like an electrocuted version of Phyllis Diller, they had no choice.

Tommy did the first round and Brandon finished it up with a hot shave. I have to hand it to them both; they did a spanking good job (if your goal is to be bald). They understood my reasoning but I could see in their faces that it hurt them to see me like that. It's not the hair, per se, it's that I now looked the part. I looked *just like a chemo patient.*

The dog freaked out. I could have done without that. For two days she would not let me touch her, instead she tucked her tail between her legs and scurried away, casting me dirty looks in route.

From there on everyone felt duty bound to assess my head (the few people who saw me) and tell me that I have a beautifully shaped head. This, to me, is like telling me that my chicken laid a very nice egg. I suppose it beats hearing that I look like Uncle Fester, but it still does not make me Sinead O' Connor or Iman. And no one who is outside of my house will ever know what my head looks like anyway because it is FREEZING and I have become one with my hats. Long live the beanie! This is what I get for doing all this in the winter. I briefly pointed this out to Terminal, trying to blame him, but he immediately rallied that it was this or a sunburnt head and that shut me right on up.

At first I was really OK with it. I remember quite clearly getting out of the shower, very pleased with myself for "handling" this and not letting vanity play a part in my life.

This is where Terminal just loooooooves to jump in and throw curve balls at me.

"You do realize that this means you are going to lose ALL your hair, don't you?"

One would think that, by now, I would learn to think before I just knee-jerk fire back at him, but I'm not sure I ever will. I don't have the advantage of full sight like he does and he just flat out *enjoys* giving me my lessons piecemeal. I suppose it is similar to how one deals with a male that needs to do something, but has to *believe* they are the one who *came up* with the idea.

"So what, Terminal? I lose my pubic hair, I no longer have to shave my legs and armpits, Poor pitiful me. I can live with that. If I need to look decent, I'll throw some mascara on."
"On what?" Point Terminal.

OMG! I'm going to lose my eyebrows and my eyelashes!?!! This had not occurred to me! I stared at myself in the mirror for a while, trying to envision this scenario. I finally told myself it didn't matter anyway because I do not subscribe to vanity.

This is such a crock of shit it's laughable (as fairly demonstrated by Terminal). Sitting in the doctor's office being told that I may *not* lose my hair after all was a clear indication of how important it is to me NOT to lose my hair and how much I *hate* being bald. Now I have taken to washing my Velcro with "growth enhancing" shampoo and such behaviors.

Yes, it *matters* to me now. And yes, I am a hypocrite. If the truth be known most of that was born of sheer laziness. My hair was unruly as hell, and blow drying and all that business is time consuming and boring to me, so.... brush the stuff and put it up with a pen while attributing this lack of self-care to a much higher quality known as the "free spirit" who is unencumbered by the trappings of vanity and pride.

Like I said, what a crock of shit.

"You're so vain, you probably think this song is about you, don't you, don't you?"

Oh my God. He's singing.

"Stop with the singing already!"

I *could* blame Carly Simon and the song, "You're So Vain," which resonated through my formative years, but I am pretty sure she is not the culprit. That belongs to my mother.

Now I'm ready to launch into that bit of self-exploration (which really isn't the point of this little book) but I feel strongly inclined to go into the extreme loss of weight and suddenly there is a ruckus upstairs and sure enough – SOMEBODY has arrived with an opinion on the matter.

"Hello Terminal. I heard you throwing things. Is something bothering you, perchance?"
"Yes. Why are you doing that?"
"Doing WHAT? Examining and owning my vanity? That was your brilliant idea, remember?"
Clearly exasperated, he grabs a couple handfuls of his hair and tugs on them. A trait I used to share. "Stop doing things with your hair. Now you are just showing off."
"And you are sulking. You have hair."
"Noooo, I have STUBBLE! WHAT is the problem?"
"You are being simpleminded and unfair. This is NOT your mother's fault. Don't be a bitch."
Instantly defensive, I say, "I'm not being a bitch. I'm being ACCURATE, to coin your phrase. She's already dead, Terminal, she will never read this."
He rolls his eyes in the most grandiose of manners and accents the show with a heaving sigh. Then he affects that "tone." His tone is one of a very wise adult trying his best to be patient with a small child and explain what he considers to be the obvious. "I apologize for my frustration. It's just that I consider you to be smarter than this. Your mother is the obvious answer, but you are not considering what got HER there. What got her there, Sharon?"
"My Grandmother?"
So much for the exaggerated patience. "DAMMIT SHARON! DON'T BE SO FUCKING OBTUSE! You know that most women have chronic insecurities – you have spent the better part of your CAREER helping women get through these insecurities! Did you all have the same MOTHER??!!"

In an instant I knew *exactly* what he was talking about.

Obtuse? *Obtuse*!?!! Nobody has *ever* called me "obtuse" before.

I'm used to being called "smart." My pride was hurt, I realized, and just kind of collapsed at that point. If my poor pride gets hurt anymore it's going to wither and die.

I needed a minute to reflect.

My mother was *very* vain. She firmly believed that her only worth was her beauty – and she was, until her dying day, *exceptionally* beautiful. She was equally intelligent, conniving, manipulative as needed, perfectly coiffed, well versed in *everything*, well educated and capable. But she was also firmly convinced that the most *important* thing about her was her appearance and her ability to attract and "catch" a man. That is what she saw as her self-worth. You can't be too thin or too tall or too pretty. We were taught to walk with books on our heads, for chrissakes. People love my hands. Like my mother, I have gnarled hands – but she spent HOURS teaching us to move them by leading with our wrists (I'm sooo ready and primed to be a Rose Queen Parade Princess you would not believe it) so that they give the illusion of being pretty. I could go on and on. I was tall, dark, thin and pretty. And I have very long legs, to boot! She had great hopes for me – I was surely going to attract one of those nice Stanford Boys they invited over for these ridiculous dinners – and all her future financial worries would be solved.

Unfortunately for her, I was also an artist, rebellious, independent and opinionated. Suffice it to say that I failed miserably at seducing a doctor.

So one can see where it would be easy enough for me to put all this on my mother. But Terminal was right to call me obtuse, although I think he could have been a little more diplomatic. Mom was merely the messenger. And pinning all of my bullshit on her, dead or alive, is pretty much as empty as vanity itself. She was merely ONE of the messengers.

It didn't come from my grandmother either. It came from Society. And it still does.

My mother was born in 1933. In her youth skirts got shorter, cigarettes were now OK for the ladies, and some even indulged with a nip or two of the hard stuff. WWII taught women that they could work, be independent to a *point* – everything changed then. But it all had the underlying message – be sexy, be beautiful, but do not think for one *second* you have the value of a man. Your job is to *seduce* and *support*.

Soooo many women in that generation that I know, particularly out here in California, suffer from the same influences and have unwittingly passed them along.

And they had help from the media. *Lots* of help. It started for my generation with "Young Miss" magazine, where we learned about tanning oils, lip gloss, the importance of pink fingernails, and other pertinent stuff. It went on from there.

So, rather than admit to any vanity, I took my God-given looks for granted (don't do that – they are so short lived) and pronounced myself "above" mortal vanity. My camera saved me for a long time because it was then my job to photograph the beauty in another and what I looked like did not matter two shakes to the end result.

I let myself go in *fear*. In fear that I might become superficial, that I might intimidate someone else. I was tired of being hurt by my own mirror that kept getting older. I discounted my own appearance completely, living through the world around me visually, sure that I would never be good enough and it morphed right into some caricature of what I used to look like.

What-I-Look-Like-Doesn't-Matter had turned into I-Don't-Care-About-Me.

In that moment at the doctor's office when I sat there gaping like a guppy, opening and closing my mouth, a little bit of self-pride came rushing back in. I *want* my hair back. I *want* to have some vanity again. I *want* to look good again. I can get up and put on some mascara! It doesn't make me vain and horrible; it just makes me feel pretty. I can simply do it for *me*.

I have learned to put myself in the back corner. I have learned to put others first; I have learned to be compassionate and understanding. Now I just want to be pretty for one of my last minutes without feeling guilty. Damnit hair – GROW!

Terminal had just taught me moderation. And he was *still* singing upstairs.

Yep, I was living with the earworm from hell.

10. THE PORT

This is rather weird to say, but I've always been proud of my veins. I have good veins. They are front and center and when it is time for someone to stick a needle in them, they behave just *fine*. That was then and this is now. Some years prior to all of this, I had a partial mastectomy (lumpectomy). This is no big deal but on account of them grabbing a few lymph nodes for testing I can't let them go messing around with the veins on that side. This has never presented a problem, until *now*. Chemo drips and blood draws are not the same thing. And very quickly your veins get tired of the whole game and flat out *hide*.

In other words, they go MIA. When they are finally found it hurts like holy hell. I was shocked to hear myself yelling in pain on chemo two.

So much for good veins. Once I was done with my other dramatic episode of that day, several of the other patients told me to go get the port, promising me that I would be glad I did and that it was no big deal.

So off I go to the hospital to have this little "procedure" done.

*"Why do they call this a 'procedure' and not a surgery?" I asked
Terminal.*
*"Because they aren't putting you completely under and you don't
have to spend the night."*
*"Sounds to me like they are just selling me a sack of goods.
Anytime they are cutting someone open and inserting a foreign
object into them, it is surgery."*
*"But 'procedure' makes it sound like so much less to worry about,
don't you think?"*

No. But then I *am* a worrier. That is just how I roll.

Oddly enough, however, this time I wasn't anywhere as nervous
about it as I would have been before all this. Hell, I have been
through so much by this time that the idea of getting knocked out
for a couple hours didn't bother me in the slightest. But they
weren't knocking me out *completely*. I took that to mean they were
going to give me the pre-anesthesia drugs that kind of put you in
zombie land where you don't care about much. Fine. That works
too.

The actual procedure, it turns out, only takes about 15 minutes.
The reason I had to be there for a couple of hours was so that I
could read magazines in my cute little hospital gown and wait. As
usual for this kind of thing, I was not allowed to eat or drink after
midnight the night before.

And, as usual, this sudden restriction has me hungry as hell,
eyeballing my neighbor's untouched apple juice and trying really
hard not to think about food.

"All I can think about is bacon."
*"Seriously? You never eat breakfast anyway. Why is this such a
big deal all of a sudden?"*
*"Because I am STARVING, Terminal! I can't believe my stomach
isn't growling!"*
*"No.... your stomach doesn't need to growl. You are doing a fine
job of that on your own. Stop complaining."*

I quit growling then and substituted it with a nice hiss instead. He took the point and left me thinking about tapioca pudding and staring at the food ads in the magazine.

In fairly short order, some nice young man came to get me. Into the operating room we went. They moved me to my bed and he got me sorted out with some covering on my head with a little window. Time passed and I waited to go into never-never land. It didn't happen.

What did happen, *however*, was that I was treated to a fascinating, albeit terribly frustrating, conversation, between the doctor, the surgical nurse, and my nurse. All about *food*. Who is bringing what to Thanksgiving dinner, who has a great recipe for sweet potatoes, and which stuffing is better – sausage or oyster?

REALLY?

"Oyster stuffing sounds gross."
"You can't eat, can you?"
"Well, no. But it still sounds gross. What kind of stuffing do you make?"
"Sausage. Is this really necessary? You aren't helping, you know."
"Yes I am too! I'm distracting you!"
"From what? Food? Can't say you are doing a spectacular job of that, Terminal."
"No, not from food, from the procedure at hand."

At that point I felt a little thumping on my chest. Like you would feel if you took your fingers and went tap, tap, tap. I guessed he was checking for placement and any minute they would give me the meds. I decided to check in.

"Hey guys! Remember me? The woman on the table who hasn't eaten since yesterday?"

"Yes! Hello! You are here!"

Laughing, I said, "Yes I am! Can I make a request for a topic change? I'm about ready to eat my little tent right about now. When are we going to start by the way?"

"Start? I just *finished*!"

The nurse took my tent off to protect it from some obscure carnivorous attack and *lo and behold*, we were all done! I looked down at my newly-installed alien and off we went to recovery. My nurse got me onto the bed and within seconds manifested both the worst and the best chicken salad sandwich I had ever had.

"Sorry it isn't oyster stuffing", he says with a wry smile. And then I went home.

I don't know if they ever gave me anything or not, to tell you the truth. It was sore for a few days, but no big deal. The scariest part of the day was my husband running amok with our credit cards for two hours unsupervised.

In other words? Just go get the damn port.

11. THE BLESSING AND THE CURSE

"Terminal, is this a blessing or a curse?"

He was in his lounge chair, supine in his forever-casual glory, with his cap tilted over his head in such a way as to lead someone to believe he was asleep. I didn't know if he was or not, but this little shit had interrupted my sleep so many times, I really didn't care if I woke him up.

Once again, he is ahead of me. Without raising his head, he says,
"I've NEVER interrupted your sleep. Never."
"Really? Because I'm up several times a night."
"Talk to your bladder. That isn't my department." Back to feigning
sleep.
"My question still stands."
"It's both. Sometimes it takes one to find the other. The answer to
your question is: Ultimately it's your call."

Dammit. Dammit. *Dammit.* I went back down to my quarters and thought about this. It's so true. It's *profoundly* true, actually. It's been true my whole life, if I think about it, but certainly not quite as obvious as it is at this juncture.

Our whole lives are about choices, or that is what they *tell* us. Of course, they tell us that when we are somewhere between looking for love in all the wrong places and looking for trouble. It resonates, but when someone tries to tell a poor single mother who is writing newspaper columns for $20 each and driving the newspaper up to be printed in the middle of the night for another whole $20, scrubbing someone else's bathroom with a baby strapped to her or whatever, that this is all *her choice*, is, well, ludicrous at *best*. Yes. You *caught* me. I admit it; I CHOSE this life. I would advise against saying that to younger people. But it *is* true. We have choices to make. And we don't always do a good job with that. If you think you are exempt from this, take a good look at the list of people you "dated". Uh-huh. I'm going to go out on a limb here and suggest that they were not always the most *stellar* of choices. But as we get older, unstrap the babies (ha! Like that ever really happens!) and look around, we can start to see it. Our insecurities become less veiled, and we start to *try*. My 30's and 40's were mainly about that. Still a lot of I'm-the-victim stuff, but also seeing that I *did* have choices. I wasn't just living out some pre-scripted play all the time. Sometimes, yes. But in my 50's I learned (slowly), that while not everything that affects me is something of my own *choosing*, how I deal with it is *all mine*. Getting the damn cancer wasn't my choice, unless that happened *before* I got here and I just don't remember drawing out the "grand plan" before I came into the world, but ever since I got my diagnosis it's been *one big choice.*

Am I going to focus on *living* or am I going to focus on *dying*? That, right there, is my choice.

Sounds easy enough, but it isn't quite that straightforward. What happens is that your whole life comes into very sharp focus. Every nuance, every relationship, every movement. It's right there in your face. POW! All of it at once. We are not equipped for this – to sort all this in nanoseconds is impossible.

Add chemo brain to the equation, and you don't know which end is up and all you are left with are fragments of a puzzle you have to try and put together while you are bewildered, angry, and

71

confused. It's very weird. And you have no time in which to do it because you are *terminal*. And your clock is ticking. Loudly. Should I make little refrigerator magnets with pictures of me to be handed out at my funeral? Should they say "Thank you" or should they say "You will be fine without me, suck it up." THAT is what my life immediately separated into. Right out of the gate. Every one of my human interactions became crystal clear to me, as though someone had washed a window for the first time. (Well, not "someone"; I knew who. The same clown who was snoring in his recliner upstairs). At first, I found myself reeling out of control, bombarded by horrific moments of clarity. So many people, SOOO many people were only engaged in themselves and what I could give them. The sobbing, the carrying on, with little or no regard toward me and how I was feeling. I was bombarded with unbelievable comments such as, "I can't talk about this. I can't talk to you. What am I going to do without you? I can't face this, who am I going to talk to *now*?" *Seriously* people?

Here I was, just trying to let those whom I considered good friends know and too often I found myself wanting to scream, "Well, excuse the fuck out of me! I guess you can just go out and PAY to have someone listen to you now!" I felt deserted, disappointed, shocked.

I felt alone.

Really alone.

And I felt like a fool. Why didn't I see these people for who they really were? Why had I dedicated so much of my time and energy to some of these people? It was like falling into a black hole, desperately reaching out for someone's hand to grab me and pull me up, yet so many people were too worried about themselves to bother. Why was this so paramount in my mind? Why did this hurt me so *much*?

Mercifully this did not extend to *everyone* in my life, certainly not to my husband nor to my sons. Ironic when one stops to realize that they are the ones who really *will* lose something when I go. Thankfully, I have made it as far as 61 in my life which has lent me a *little* bit of self-restraint and wisdom, if not a lot. I had the sense to know that I was going insane on some level so I went completely underground until I could think. I spoke to no one for over a month.

By that time, I thought I had it pretty well under wraps. I didn't *need* to talk to most of these people. I needed to be courteous and refrain from a select number of comments and reactions, but it was easy enough to avoid conversation for the most part and I rested knowing that most of them would slip away of their own accord without me there to breastfeed them whenever they felt they needed it.

And I *needed* to dive inside myself. I'm astonished at how much of my life I have spent dedicated to the care and feeding of people who are, essentially, self-absorbed walking insecurity attacks. It must be my compassionate nature?

Terminal informed me that I was being too kind to myself with that. (No one has ever accused *him* of excessive kindness, I assure you of that much). And I guess he is right. Upon further introspection, I have come to realize that what I was doing/creating was largely due to my *own* insecurities. If I could fill my time with all of that, I wouldn't have to spend my time reaching into the things that I "wanted" to do – expand my career, write my books, paint again–and not be such a coward about putting these things out into the world. Can't blame myself if my avoidance tactics are "helping" others, right? I had to face it: *I had chosen these people as an excuse not to face my own fear of success.*

Lies. I've been deluding myself and wasting time with my own pack of lies. I hate it when people lie to me and, here I was, *lying to myself.* Spectacular, Sharon!

Once I realized *that* I began to find some balance and temperance. First, I had to realize that I had put expectations on a number of people who are simply incapable of fulfilling them. It's not their fault, they simply don't get anything outside of their own universe. And they really don't want to. They get comfortable and complacent and addicted to being a victim, unable or unwilling to change that. Simpleminded souls and here comes the eminently "wise" one to be a good listener and proffer advice that a five-year-old could give. I'm such a rock star.

I got sick of them first and sick of *me* right after that.

In the beginning I was too harsh. Too quick. And, if the truth be told, downright *mean*. I have a shit-ton of excuses, of course, all valid, but *still*.

Time goes on though. I'm learning that today's truth means absolutely *nothing* tomorrow. I've made a few humble apologies, touting aforementioned and socially correct excuses. I'm finding that I miss people. A lot. I don't need to stand in judgment, but by the same token, I don't need to make myself available for everyone else's problems *first*. I am not a bad guy if I choose not to go down a one-way street anymore. But I *am* innately kind and I *do* care and if someone needs me, I feel that now I can make a more balanced determination of whether or not I can afford to expend that energy without it being to my detriment. I hope like hell this isn't "too little, too late."

Maybe that is what it means when they say, "Take care of yourself."

So there it is. I've put expectations on people that are downright unfair. Yes, it has left me disappointed in so many places, but am I? Really? Do I even *like* these people? I like having playmates, having dinner, going on trips, the simple things, and I like having people to do that with. But when I look at how much effort I put into making those "friendships" a reality and those people walked away when I wasn't *fun* anymore... Well, I am ashamed of myself. It's shocking.

If I learn anything from this, I hope I can learn to be more discriminating. Not judgmental, but to recognize that these are not people who have anything to bring to my particular life. I have no time to waste anymore. With whatever I have left, time-wise, I want to fill it with people who can spark my interest in something, people who bring something to my table, not people who only come for what they can get. All of this was and still is my choice.

Damn. I am an idiot.

From upstairs I hear someone say "*BINGO!*" I hope that he was referring to my insight, but I highly suspect that he was referring to my last sentence.

12. CHEMO NUMBER THREE

I was in for a long day this time and so was my nurse. On chemo 2 she had to forgo a dinner date with her boyfriend who had been gone for some time, all in the name of keeping me alive. (No she did not whine about this, I found it out accidentally.) Since I know she is a foodie, I brought my shrimp pasta for everybody. I love to feed people.

I was tra la la about the whole thing until I got in the chair. My heart started racing. Then I remembered the last time. OH MY GOD, I'M GONNA DIE!

"Yes, you idiot, if you keep this shit up, you are going to die.of Paranoia Cancer. Bully for you. Why this time?"
"My heart is racing.'
"No shit Sherlock – it's knocking my stuff off the shelves and my favorite bean bag chair bounced over and got wedged under my console. Stop already."
"Trust me on this – I'm trying."
"What is the problem NOW?"
"I'm afraid I will go back to that shock thing and it will kill me."
"Oh, for the love of God, woman, it isn't going to kill you!"
"I thought that was your goal, how can I trust you on this?"

And here comes the exasperated sigh of the overly patient tone again. "I am not Death. I am a Diagnosis. My goal isn't to kill you and see you die. How many times do I have to explain this to you?"
"Try once. Pretty sure you haven't explained anything to me. Do you even KNOW what 'explaining' means?"

He mumbles something; pretty sure I heard the words "such a bitch," but I ignored it.

"OK. I am here as a slap in the face, if you will. My job is to find out what you really want and how far you are willing to go to get that. But in order to do that, I have to push you into realizing who you truly are and what you truly want, because – and trust me on this – if you don't figure that out you cannot stave off the Big Guy. So far, I think you want to live. Not everyone does, you know. So, try not to kill the middleman, OK?"

My heart was still racing and now my mind along with it. Kerrylea came over to check me. "I think it's anxiety," she says, "I can give you something for that." I am always suspicious of a new pill. "Have you ever had Ativan?" No. I haven't. I have a whole bottle of it at home but I had no idea why it was prescribed to me and therefore I have never taken one. She assures me it will help. And away we go!

Holy shit. I was high as a kite in thirty seconds and out like a light thirty seconds after that. I guess that's ONE way to deal with anxiety – just go into a *coma.*

I drink wine. I admit it, I *love* my wine, but the nice thing about wine is that I know where I am at and when to stop. This was twenty-five bottles of GOODNIGHT IRENE!

However, the bladder wakeup call is stronger than *any drug known to man.* I'm awake now and I have to pee. I unplug Mr. Stick from the wall and make my way towards the restroom. All I can say is thank God for Mr. Stick. (The roll around thing that holds the IV bags and beeps a lot). I could barely walk. I knew the bathroom was straight ahead and the door was on the right. HOWEVER, my legs had their *own* plan and I found myself in the nurse's station looking *across* their desk at the suddenly illusive bathroom door. This was seriously *not* the plan. After I pointed this out to my body, my legs got me out of there and towards the storage room. Nooooo... U turn guys, U turn! We managed that much as a team and, *somehow,* I got all the way to the toilet and *somehow* back to my chair. Then I slept for another three hours.

What IS this stuff? When I *finally* woke up, Kerrylea informed me that I only had an hour to go. Good gravy. It was like being under anesthesia. Just blank, except for my bladder who wanted to make sure I was still alive, apparently. I don't like to fly, but if I ever have to go overseas again, I know *my* drug of choice!

When I went back up for my shot the next day, Kerrylea asked me if I even *remembered* yesterday. I told her no, except standing in front of her desk and wondering if I was going to wind up peeing in her file cabinet drawer.

Sooo... there is chemo three for you. I guess I could play the anxiety card again next time, but I was kind of bummed. It was like I missed the whole experience of the people around me. I missed part of my *life*. Now THAT is weird. One would think that you would want to just go in, get knocked out and go home. But...but....but...there's other *people* to see and meet if only for a second, right? It's my *new* life! I don't want to *sleep* through it!

"Don't you worry about that. Believe me that they knew you were there. You snored the entire five hours."
"Oh no. Did I really?"
"Yes ma'am, you sure did. It was great sport."
"So glad you could have some fun at my expense."
"I always have fun at your expense. Nobody cared anyway. At least it was a break from the babbling."
"I'm so embarrassed."
"Cheer up; at least no one told you that you have sleep apnea!"

Suddenly Terminal

It was after the chemo treatment that this got noteworthy.

This was number three of six, providing my body would hold up for six; apparently most people didn't make it after four. There are a myriad of reasons for that, I presume. However, when the doctor first told me that I thought it was because the chemo was so hard they simply jumped ship on it. Now I know that it has more to do with blood cells. But so far I was OK there.

I saw the doctor for a checkup. I was feeling pretty darn good, so I dressed nicely for once. He was very impressed. I thought it was my stellar dress style and the mascara (I still had lashes), but that wasn't what he saw. He saw color in my face, heard me laughing, although he did say that the pearls were a nice touch. He told us that he *knew* the chemo was working and he didn't feel that he even needed to do any tests. While this made me feel great, I wasn't happy with just a handshake. I needed the contract. Show it to me on paper, baby!

Off they sent me for a CT scan, and, as usual, more blood draws. I go back to the doc for the results and he tells me it all looks good like he "knew" it would. Smile.

Uh, define "good" please.

"Everything is shrinking".

Define "everything" please.

Holy shit. I don't think I wrapped my head around it when he told me the cancer was "everywhere." I was in shock. A little after the fact, mind you, but in shock, nonetheless. Jesus! No *wonder* everything hurt!

"The good news is that your markers are down to 3200!" He says jubilantly. He may as well have been talking to me in Klingon. I haven't the *slightest* idea what he is talking about. Not a bloody clue.

I stare at him blankly. "What is a marker and what does it do?"

He explained that these are cancer markers that count the number of cancer cells in my body. And? *What?*

I knew about white blood cell count, and I knew big numbers were my friend in *that* department, but I kinda doubted that it worked the same way with "cancer markers" and 3200 sounded pretty big to me! Desperately wanting me to join in with his celebratory enthusiasm, he told me that I had lost 7000 whatever-they-ares, having come in well over 10,000 to start.

For me this was your classic glass-half-empty kind of deal. Tommy seemed pretty happy, high-fiving me out the door, but I didn't get it. 3200 wasn't zero! But then, zero probably wouldn't have done it for me *either*. One year prior, I was declared cancer free and nine months later I rolled back in with stage 4 metastatic cancer and only a couple months to live.

"For the love of all things holy, woman, what is your problem NOW?" Terminal was leaning against a door, smoking a cigar, he had a new jacket and hat.
"Nothing. Clearly chemo is working and that's all I can hope for, right? I'm happy."
"And you are lying. Again, you are not Superwoman. Did you expect it all to be gone with only half the treatments?" He paused and took a drag off his cigar, "You DID, didn't you?"
"No, I 'hoped' it would. But I'm happy. It's working anyway."
"Have you ever been happy? I mean really happy, not just satisfied?"
"Sure I have."

I flashed back to one time in particular. It was shortly after we finally got married. I was standing on my back porch of my newly rebuilt house (fire) and just overwhelmed by how very blessed and happy I was. Two weeks later they found my first cancer (breast.) And I've been happy since then, but it seems very much like the minute I let myself feel that way another bomb drops. And I'm not talking about *little* bombs. I am talking about *big* bombs. Death and cancer. So, yeah, maybe a part of me is afraid to be too happy.

"Why?" (I forget he can read my thoughts if he is so inclined – after all, he lives in my brain.) "Is that because you think if you are really happy you are going to suffer another big loss and 'pay' for that moment of happiness?"
I looked at him, all cavalier in his new digs, looking for all the world like some short movie star out of a 1950's movie gone bad. "Yes. I think so."
"That's because you don't believe you deserve it. You think you will be made to pay for it. Did it ever occur to you that that line of thinking is sheer arrogance?"
"It is NOT!"
"Actually, it is," he takes another drag of the cigar and blows a smoke ring, all for dramatic effect. I know he wanted me to, but I wasn't about to conjure up a vision of a street lamp at night on a dark street with mist. Nope. Not doing it. "Basically you are saying that people die for your happiness."
"I most certainly am NOT!"
"Yes, you are. You are saying that the universe is going to either punish you with cancer or kill off your friends if you are happy."
Damn. "Cancer, just so you know, is not an entity of its own. It's more like a dumb slug that just burrows around. Death I know quite well. He comes for someone when THEIR time is up. He's pretty matter-of-fact and seldom open to negotiation. Negotiation is my job, Sharon. Death is less personal. Someone else's death is not about you. You complain about people trying to make your cancer about them when it's not, well...isn't this the same thing?"

I looked at him. For once I didn't want to smack him. He was spot on.

"Where did you get the jacket anyway?" (When guilty, change the subject, right?)
"Do you like it? Don't you recognize it? You used to wear it all the time."
Well, I'll be jiggered. It's my grandfather's jacket and I used to

wear it all the time.

"You have a whole thrift store of cool shit in here, girl!"

"I have a WHAT?"

"A thrift store. Well, I call it that, but it's a room in your brain where you have kept things that you no longer have, but used to love. Things that you felt good in, or that made a statement. Memories. You have some great memory clothes here, I have to say!"

"Really?" This is fascinating to me. "What else?"

"How about this hat?"

I cringed a little at that one. I had a big head and hats were all the rage when I was thirteen. All the cool girls would try on hats in the girls' section, but I had to go to the men's department to find anything that fit me.

"How about my jeans with the paint on them?"

"Right here, baby. Check these bad boys out!" He held up my favorite 501s. It was so cool.

I smiled then. And I kept smiling all day. I only had three more chemo treatments to go, and I was making headway. I could own that. "Happy" wasn't punishable by divine law after all!! *Who knew?*

"You oughta try on some of my dresses from back in the day. I had some pretty good stuff; you would look good in it!"

I left him choking on his cigar.

13. WEIGHING IN

While there are exceptions to this, as with anything, most people lose weight with chemotherapy. Now, this is not a diet that I would personally *recommend*, and for God's sake don't say something stupid to your chemo friend like, "Oh, I'm so jealous, I wish I could lose weight like that" and be within arm's reach or that skinny chick might surprise you with sudden agility and strength.

While it sounds great on the surface, and trust me, I had plenty of excess to spare – it's alarming when it happens. Because it happens *fast*.

Now I am not going to lie to you – there was a part of me that took pleasure in seeing the numbers go down. At first. There are two reasons for this – one is that my particular type of cancer (Endometrial Cancer Gone Haywire) creates fluid in your stomach. And I'm not talking about a full bladder here – I'm talking ten months pregnant with twins. No exaggeration. And along with *that* comes all the pain and discomfort of carrying said twins. Times 500. They would drain me (*liters* at a time) but within ten days I needed to do it again. But as the cancer receded, so did that crap. That was *very* encouraging.

The other part of me was full-on Vain Female. I was always a tall, thin woman until my 50's when I blew up like a *tick*. So – while

YOU, who do *not* have cancer, are *not* allowed to say this to US who *do* have cancer – YIPEEEE! BRING IT BABY!!! I'll take whatever perks I can get!

This works for a minute.

I went into this at 184 pounds. Four weeks later I was 154. I was thrilled with that. Lots of it was fluid, and I no longer looked like I was having a *baby*.

Eight days later I was 143. I was *not* thrilled with that. It wasn't the number that got me, per se. 143 is fine for me. But 133 isn't and certainly not 123. *One week?* 11 pounds in *one week?* I was sure they had screwed up. I made them weigh me three times and finally started to cry. I'm eating! I'm eating A LOT! I have four or five days right after chemo where it's not so much – but the rest of the time I'm a regular chowhound. And stuff I've avoided for years! You ought to see me devour the fat on the edge of a steak! What the *hell*?

I was terrified. I had only done three treatments so far out of six. What if this kept up? Would I wind up all alone in a hospital on a damn feeding tube?

Mercifully, my doctor assured me the bulk of this was due to the diuretic they gave me. (My legs and feet had blown up in keeping with my new pregnant look).

I'm near the end and holding around 145. I'm OK with that.

"Be honest. You are more than OK with that. You like that."
And here he is again, back by popular demand, it's Terminal!
"Well, Hello! Here you are invading my personal thoughts again. Can't you just keep your opinions to yourself for once?"
"No", says Everybody's Unwanted Houseguest.
"And why not?"
"Because I am PART of your thoughts. I exist in your mind; you created me."

"That's just fabulous. I'm dying AND insane!"
"Get over it. You have always had an imaginary friend. Ever since you were little. And hey! At 143 you are little again, so why not? Go with the flow."
"If you are imaginary then does that mean I'm not terminal and dying?"
"I don't know. You tell me."
"SERIOUSLY? Listen, Mr. Figment, if I created you, that means I can un-create you, right?"
I meant this to be snarky and retaliatory. His answer surprised me.
"Yup. But you don't know HOW yet. That is what we are working on. So why don't you be honest with yourself and enjoy your body for once without constantly finding fault with it? Go shopping. Get out of those wretched sweatpants. Do something. Stop hiding."

Once again Terminal has cut straight to the chase. I wonder if he is truly of my own invention and not some divine (HA!) little critter that somehow floated in. In other words, why don't I have that kind of clarity without being diagnosed as dying?

I *did* need to go shopping, it was true: 40 pounds in a couple months is an awful lot to lose, and nothing fits me. *Nothing.* But it didn't really matter as I had been living in beater sweat pants and my husband's old T-shirts for a very long time. Who cares, *right*? Well, suddenly *I* cared. I went to my closet.

Prior to this whole nightmare, I had gone clothes shopping for the first time in YEARS. I was headed for a vacation with my two younger sisters who are both athletes and, well, *perfect.* For several days prior to this I worked on my psyche. I had come to grips with my age and the simple fact that I am this weight, I'm probably not going to change as the mere idea of a sit-up gives me the shivers. I'm just going to get a few things I feel comfortable in and are presentable in public. With the help of a friend, I did it and we had a blast. I actually came home with some lovely clothes. I pulled out one of these outfits and put on the fabulous, EXPENSIVE, palazzo pants. Straight down. A slight hesitation at the hips and then bye-bye. See ya! To the ground they went.

SUDDENLY TERMINAL

Shit.

I found I could wear my jeans with a belt and one pair wasn't too bad. That was something, anyway. A start.

Next came a bra. I hadn't been able to wear a bra in months due to all the fluid and having to wear a brace, etc. I put on my bra. I used to be a healthy DD; since I was 20. My bras are great. They are somewhat molded and hold their shape (Bali bras for those of you who are looking). I put it on. OK! Then I look down.

The bra is holding form just fine, but it is all alone, apparently. I look down to where my breast *should* be puffing out and all I see is a dark, empty cavern about three inches wide off the top of my ribcage with some sort of fleshy puddle down at the bottom.

"OH MY GOD! What is *this* now?!!!" In desperation I plunge my cold hand down into the mausoleum-formally-known-as-my-bra and hoist up one of the girls. I release her and watch her plop right back down to the bottom of the cavern with a sigh. The sigh was barely audible due to the giggling.

"Terminal? This isn't funny."
"Yes, it is. Admit it. You are standing there asking your boob where the rest of her got to and, well, this is hilarious, frankly. C'mon, admit it – this is FUNNY. What did you expect? Dolly Parton revisited?"
"Why not?"

But I did have to laugh. My husband was never a big boob guy anyway. Now, if he can find them somewhere much closer to my waist, he ought to be happy.

I lamented all this to a girlfriend who has never been chesty and sports the forever cute perky boobs and she told me this was a great thing! I didn't *need* a bra – just a cute little camisole and a couple fitted tank tops under my shirts. And in her world this is true. But as I told her, there is a big difference between the boob that never got big in the first place and the now deflated Hindenburgs. Trust me; *seriously not the same.*

After that I braved standing naked in front of the mirror. I've got a new body, after all.

Boy howdy do I ever! I stood there trying to absorb this "new" body. Sure didn't look "new" to me. In fact, it looked rather "old."

"What is it?'
"You are the mind reader, you tell me!"
"It's the upper arms, isn't it?"
"What the hell happened to my muscle tone?"

My upper arms had become just like my mothers about 20 years too soon. You know the arms: Saggy, wobbly and covered with long, loose skin? Apparently, it was *not* muscle tone that was keeping those together, it was *fat*. Now I have *deflated* fat. And, upon closer inspection, I have inner thighs to match.

"You ARE 60, you know."
"Yup. I'm pretty clear on that. 61, actually".
"And a half!"
"Is that supposed to be helpful?"
"Well, more of an excuse, so yes! Weight distribution changes with age. What are you going to do?"
"Buy my next swimsuit from the Mennonites?"

We both laughed at that. My whole world is new, and apparently that includes my body.

So, shopping it is. Tommy and I booked a room in Nevada City to make a mini-vacation of it. I was pretty excited to be able to go and try on clothes and feel good about myself. Not just stand there and be "satisfied", but to actually feel GOOD! This was an experience I don't know that I have *ever* had, to be honest. There was always something between me and that – I was too thin, too fat (even when I wasn't), had no butt, too much stomach, too tall, something – always *something*.

Dammit, I'm done with that noise. At least I still have a body. At least that body is capable of shopping again and at least I have enough hope for my future that I actually give a damn.

Off we go. First order of business was JCPenney's for a bra and whatever. I grab some bras and some jeans. I know mine are too loose but not dramatically so, so I grab a size smaller. We all love that, *right*? Just being brave enough to even TRY a size smaller is cool. These were size six. For reasons I do not understand, I had it in my head that I was a size eight before. *Denial is a beautiful thing.*

I get into the coldest dressing room in America and strip down to my panties. Bra first.

The D doesn't work. The C doesn't work. Holy shit, I'm a B? Well, that explains at least 12 pounds of the weight loss.

Then I go for the jeans. I had pulled a pair of "skinny" jeans because, why not? I have long and proportionately thin legs, so…. I pull them on. They fit great on my *legs*.

Then I am in trouble. Big trouble, right here in the dressing room. As I figured it might behoove me to have my pants up *over* my hips and covering the more private part of my body instead of just rolled over to my now-stuck-together legs, I needed to take them off. *This is clearly not the size for me.*

Right away I am in trouble. The problem is my feet. I'm not short and neither are my feet. Skinny jeans, I learned, have two-inch circumferences on the ankles apparently. I do the step-on-the-pant leg with one foot and pull-the-other-foot game several times and while one leg is no longer *glued* to the other, I'm still shackled. I can't easily bring my foot up to a reachable point and SHIT! Next thing I know I am on the floor of the dressing room, on my back, flailing about like some long-legged turtle on its back, desperately trying to capture my airborne foot and muscle my way out of these god-forsaken, albeit cute, jeans. I considered calling Tommy, but I was not sure I needed the hysterical laughing nor did I want to live through the social ramifications of what I knew was the perfect photo op.

Eventually I won the war, crawled back to the bench, pulled myself up and sat there panting. At least I was no longer cold. Completely frustrated and having had more physical exercise than I have had in *years*, I grabbed my old jeans and looked at the tag. Shit. I wasn't an *eight*, I was a *twelve*! These are a *six*.

"You are really good at lying to yourself, aren't you?"
"And you are really LOUSY at helping a girl out, aren't you, Terminal?"
"I'm a mental entity, not a physical entity. What would you have me do? Besides, I didn't want to miss the show."

At that point I was done. No more trying stuff on without help. PHYSICAL help. I took off the air-filled C bra, and simply left the dressing room leaving some sort of in-side-out denim sculpture on the floor. I figured it was a warning for future big-footed women. Tommy asks me how it went. I simply sighed in disgust (this is all his fault right now, but I can't do more than give the exasperated sigh until I figure out how, *exactly*, to blame it on *him*), stomped off back to the bras, grabbed myself a B cup, a huge puffy sweater on sale (3XXX – this fucker *will* fit!), calmed down and returned to Tommy who was standing there by the jeans.

He looks at me with the wisdom that only a long relationship can bring, "Feel better now?"

"Yes."

"I take it the jeans didn't fit?"
"You have *no* idea. But at least I have an idea of what size I am."
With that I go grab a size 8 pair of what I *think* are the same jeans.

"Don't you want to try them on?"

"Oh, *hell* no."

And off we go.

Later that day we are getting ready to go out for our evening and I brave the pants. They had better fit. I stick my leg in and my toe snags on something. Mercifully I am sitting for this event and not standing. I look. There is a hole in the jeans. Two, in fact. OMG, what did I do? They fit like a glove, I must say, but they have *holes* in them. *Pre-made* holes. Not the ones that happened naturally with our 501s but the new-fashioned ones. Hmmm. But I *like* them. They *are* cool looking. I haven't been cool looking for a long time. But I am 61.

Terminal saved me. "Look at your hair – you are just shy of a buzz cut. To hell with your age – run with the new look, woman!"

THAT was a game changer right there. I stood and looked at myself. I have a bald head, big brown eyes, and rock-star jeans. Why the hell not? Who is to say I need to look like a victim; a chemo patient? Why can't I just be some very cool old lady? Who made up the rule that we have to be a certain age to wear certain things and how did *that* get in my mind? At that precise moment I got over exposing my bald head. Suddenly I could have my *own* unique style. I ran upstairs in my mind and tried to give Termy a hug, but he was busy throwing away a bunch of my personal insecurities and just waved me off with a smile and told me to go buy big earrings.

I had so much fun on our little trip. I tried on clothes and felt *good* about myself. I took my beanie off whenever it was warm enough to do so – I still got lots of looks, but then I realized that on some level I always have, I'm noticeable – loud laugh, free-form, fun-having, wild hair, tall… I've always drawn attention. I can *work* this!

I am sick of apologizing to the world by downplaying myself and my attributes to make other people feel better about themselves and subsequently "see" me and maybe like me. I am sick and tired of apologizing for who I am to make someone else comfortable. Besides, at my age and given my prognosis, I'm rapidly running out of attributes!

Terminal taught me to look and see that I don't *need* everyone to like me. It's not that important. I need to like *myself.* And maybe if I am more me I will find people who like that person too. People who are less insecure and with whom I do not need to underplay myself to make them feel better about themselves. Maybe that all starts with a skinny body, a pair of holy jeans, a bald head and big earrings. I don't know. I don't care really, as long as it *starts.*

"You gotta start somewhere!"
"Damn straight, Terminal. Damn straight."

Side Note: When you lose weight really fast you are going to discover that you have become a *lizard.* No sunburn could peel more. I found this rather alarming, to say the least. I was sure I had developed some rare skin-eating cancer. It was then that a friend pointed out to me that I had a lot of extra skin that used to cover a lot of extra *me.* Get in the tub, soak and sluff off with a washcloth, loofah, whatever. It only takes a couple times.

14. NEW FOUND BUS PHOBIA

I swear I will throttle the very next person who says this to me: "We are all going to die *someday*. You could go out tomorrow and get hit by a bus!"

Seriously?

SERIOUSLY?

Terminal starts cracking up at that point. "Yep, it happens!"
"To two hundred and something people a year. Pretty sure I'm not going to suffer Death by Bus."
"And how do you know that?" Still snickering about the whole thing. I stopped being so mad then and regained my own sense of humor.
"Two reasons: The first one is that I am pretty sure that to get hit by a bus requires an actual BUS. I live in a town that has no damn buses. Gonna go out on a limb here and say that my probability factor is pretty damn close to zero."
"And the second reason?"
"YOU! You are the second reason. Are you going to tell me that you just suddenly show up in someone's life to let them know that they are going to be killed by a BUS in a couple months? I don't

think so."

"Well... no; not like you are thinking, but you have already realized that I am a bus of sorts and we are headed to a terminal." I had to think about that for a moment. "But YOU can't kill me. It depends on what bus is waiting for me at the end of the line, right?"

"Yes, actually, I CAN kill you."

Heart stopping moment. "What?"

"Think of it like this: If you stare too long directly into the sun, you will go blind. If you embrace me too hard and focus only on me, your soul will die and you will cease to live. Your body may still go on for a bit, but you won't be alive anymore. Strangely enough some people do this all by themselves without me even in the picture."

Holy shit. I just sat there. I was reeling. Absolutely reeling. So many thoughts; I could barely put them together. I have a huge fear of death. And I forever think I am going to be taken out. I swear, if I stub my toe, and it hurts, I think I have toenail cancer or something. It was kind of funny – a short time after my diagnosis and pre-chemo, something hurt and I thought "Oh, It's cancer!"

And a voice in my head said, *"Yes, you are right. It's cancer. You already know that. NOW what are you going to worry about? You have a big void in your thought processes to fill, girl. What is it going to be?"*

"That was the first time I talked to you and you actually heard me. You laughed because the irony of it hit you."

"That was the day I realized I had to change and there was room in my mind. I could stop punishing myself for being happy, and maybe that was the day I let my mother go. I don't know. But I decided to fill my thoughts with living thoughts."

"That was the day that you and Tommy went to see the doc for the first time and he realized that you were really dying. Do you remember what you said to him when you saw his fear?"

"Yes, actually, I do. I told him I understood it was scary that I was going to die. But that right then and right now, I just wanted to

focus on being alive. When death is at my doorstep, I would focus on dying, but not before then and not a minute before. And neither would he."

"Yep. That was it. You are a fighter; I will give you that."

"But what about the people who seem to have some burning desire to bring up this stupid 'death by bus' thing with me?"

He giggles a bit, "What about it? I, personally, like the irony. It's a no-fault-no-harm kind of thing. People aren't necessarily stupid; they just don't think. Thought is grown out of experience and, again, a choice. People learn in different ways. Or not. You made a different choice. You want to see things. Really see things. It's simply who you are. Now go to bed, will you? You are tiresome."

I AM TIRESOME? *ME*? Who has moved into whose brain and interrupts every other thought? Good gravy.

But he was right, I *was* tired and I needed to sleep. I left him to continue with his old reruns of "The Beverly Hillbillies" (He likes to sing the theme song. Mercifully it is short.)

15. CHEMO NUMBER FOUR

This one was pretty nondescript. I went in; I brought food for everyone, did my thing, and later I went home. I bounced off the ceiling for a few hours, went to bed and crashed for five days after that. But it wasn't as big a crash as before and I was happy for that. It was a routine by then. I spent two- or three-days solid watching bad Lifetime movies (I don't know why I call them bad because I *love* them), copious reruns of NCIS, and sleeping. I ate my bowls of soup, drank my protein drinks (also known as liquid chalk) and waited until I felt better. I'm living and if this is what I have to do once every three weeks to *keep* living, well then, so be it.

We had a lovely Christmas. Even Terminal was in on the gig. He surprised me with a fashion show of my favorite get-ups from my much younger years. You haven't *lived* until you see your nemesis dressed in a low-slung satin skirt, vintage chiffon shirt tied up under his man boobs, wearing more bangles and earrings than any gypsy alive, and jangling like a one-man band. He did it to make me laugh, but damn he sparked some *great* memories!

I suddenly realized that I hadn't been that free in decades. I wondered why not?

"You thought you were too fat. You grew up. You became complacent."

"I guess I did. But also, I wanted others to feel comfortable around me when I took their photographs."

"Not this again. No, you did NOT. You got lazy and used that as an excuse! You quit having fun with YOU!"

I didn't respond.

"Check this stuff out, man!" He held up another favored outfit and then my god-aw prom dress.

"Oh dear God, do not put that thing on. Pleeeease don't put that on."

He did. But he added grandpa's jacket which was a nice contrast. "HAVE SOME FUCKING FUN GIRL!!!"

"Oh, it won't last. I will be right back where I was when chemo started."

I wish I could have taken a photo. He just plopped down, right down. "Seriously? Who cares? Do YOU care? Do you have enough TIME to care? YOU who have claimed not to care what she looked like for all these years? YOU who have no problem cruising around in beat up sweatpants and her husband's T-shirts, cannot dress up in cool, fun, 'look at me' clothes for a minute? Good God, woman, WAKE UP!"

Why not, indeed! I'm officially on "borrowed time", *so why the hell not?*

I thought about what he said. When did I stop having fun with me? Don't get me wrong – I've had a hell of a lot of fun in my life. I have fun with people. I have fun with my art, my family, my garden. I'm all about fun. But I get what he is saying – I have lost my *mojo*. What *happened* to that girl in the satin skirt? The "gypsy on the loose"? Well, I got older for one thing. And I have no desire to be trucking around in that outfit now, I assure you (aside from the part where my boobs could in no way, shape or form pull that outfit off and I have no desire to see young people running in fear). There is nowhere to go now save for the grocery store and the post office. I stopped myself there. This is a newer development due to the pandemic, but I have been pulling this shit for much longer than that. *Years.*

Am I going to wait until I hit some sort of social ideal? That's impossible. So, what am I waiting for?

I *am* running out of time. Shit, for all intents and purposes I shouldn't even be standing here right now. Do I want to die without having ever put on a great outfit again? Do I need permission? If I do, who, *exactly*, is going to give me that permission? All I wanted was more days. And now I have them. Me. The answer is me.

What the hell have I been doing??????? I've been sitting here undergoing treatment, which is working, with two weeks out of three being just *fine*, my husband off work, *and...what?* Am I waiting to be "done" with this in order to go live my life again? *Why?* I have my life *right now*!

I vowed right then that I was going to start actively living. It seems like I have spent a great deal of my life waiting to accomplish this or that before I give myself the great reward of simply having *fun*. Granted, I enjoy my work, I always did, but it had a *monetary* reward which helped me justify the fun. I needed to have fun for its own sake.

That had to change. We started reaching out more to our friends, accepting invitations, and I vowed to myself that I would learn that it was perfectly OK to have fun for its own sake.

I don't know how this is all going to shake out. Every day that I feel good is a gift, and they are probably numbered. I may not be 100%, but for two out of every three weeks, I'm pretty damn good, so...here we go.

"Go get it, Tiger! I'm trying to find a Superwoman cape in here...don't you have one?
"Decidedly NOT. You may find a witch's cape, hat, and a wand, however."

"That won't work!"
"Sure it will. Haven't you seen Harry Potter?"
"Who?"
"Oh please tell me you watch something other than the Beverly Hillbillies?"
"Bonanza, but the theme song sucks."
"OK, use your imagination then. Magic. They make magic happen."
"Oh, I like that!" He disappears for a moment and returns wearing this costume. Remember he's very short and I am not. It was quite the sight to behold. "What are you doing with this stuff anyway?" He begins to jab things with the wand.
"It's a Halloween costume. And that is a WAND, not a sword. Stop poking me with it!"
"What is Halloween and what does it do?"
"Really? It's a holiday where everybody dresses up like something, mostly things related to death; skeletons, the grim reaper, stuff like that. Witches are very popular, too."
"Is it fun?"
"Yes, actually it is very fun. GIVE ME THAT!" I grab the wand out of his hand, "You WAVE it. Like this, see? You don't IMPALE people with it."
"So, this is a celebration of death, in a way."
"Sort of. Yes. In Celtic times they believed that it was the day when the veil between the dead and living was lifted and if you dressed up to look like you were already dead, or Death himself, the spirits would be more likely to leave you alone."
"And you all turned this into a party? I see. And you are worried about going out and celebrating now? Because...why, exactly? Because you don't know which side of the fence you are going to wind up on? Girl, that veil has been lifted with you for a long time now. Go celebrate living. I don't think you guys have a holiday for that, so make one."

How? *How* does he do it? I swear he can illustrate a point in the most roundabout way ever. This one was a doozy though. I went off to celebrate The Day of the Living. It's a new holiday.

98

16. HAIR REDEFINED

Just when I think it is safe to go back in the water! Just when I am so excited to have stubble, when I have accepted a moment of vanity, when I believed I had dodged the bullet.... I got hit with the bullet. Smack dab in the eyelashes.

We were meeting some friends in a cute little tourist town over the mountain for lunch and a little shopping. Yay! A day out! Some fun! I want to look nice. I finally am feeling pretty good about my bad self. I'm bald, due to my own preemptive hand, but I still have eyelashes so I head for the makeup.

Something is going very wrong with the mascara. For the life of me, I cannot get it on correctly. It's perpetually hitting my eyelid. My first line of attack is the mascara itself. I know better than to buy cheap mascara! Over and over I go through this. Granted I don't wear makeup much, but it's certainly not the first time I have applied it by any means. After rubbing it off for the fifty-seventh time, I grab the magnifying mirror and take a look. Well, well, well. This explains a lot! The reason I kept getting the mascara on my eyelid instead of my eyelashes is because I only have four eyelashes. Then I look at my eyebrows. I had noticed that they were getting increasingly lighter; closer to the color of

99

my skin. Now I saw that they were not getting lighter, they were simply 80% *gone.*

Seriously? Just when I'm getting attached to the idea of NOT losing my hair, I lose my hair?

Tommy is in the other room hollering that we need to leave. I feel tears welling in my eyes, but I won't allow it. It is what it is. My cool, new skinny jeans would have to suffice.

Off we went.

They say Bald is Beautiful. I agree that it can be on certain women. But every photo I see has the full makeup going on with it.

"Well, what about false eyelashes?"
I laugh. "The last time I put on false eyelashes one got stuck to my eyebrow and one fell off in someone's food. Besides, I don't have any".
"You have plenty of pet hair! And you have Elmer's glue – just fake it!"

Ever try to take a swing at a figment of your imagination? I gave it everything I had but could never connect with the little laughing, dodging critter.

It was a nice day – the four of us had lunch, the guys scurried off to the pub across the street and my girlfriend and I went shopping in the little boutiques along the street. It was a reasonably warm day and I took my hat off.

Bald isn't beautiful, per se, but bald is definitely *noteworthy.* I decided I was going to practice ignoring the blatant stares this time. After all, I was wearing cool earrings and cool clothes. I didn't look like a Holocaust survivor anymore. That much I was sure of. But I was remarkable, nonetheless. It was actually entertaining to see how many people snuck looks at me, but not a lot of smiles when I could catch their eyes. My head was freezing at this point, (Bald is also *cold*), but I would be damned if I would put a hat on this time. The first time I did this in public I had the beanie back on like a shot and wanted to crawl under the table for all the glares. Cancer isn't contagious people! If you are that curious and rude enough to stare, then be rude enough to trot up and ask whatever question you have. It's already an invasion of privacy, after all.

But not this time. Oh hell no. I wasn't crawling under a rock again. Not for *anyone*. I stood up tall, finished my shopping and we went to meet the guys. They got us a table and we sat down. I was hungry again, so I ordered some soup. Still no hat. I catch a lot of stares, but I'm OK with this right now. And pretty damn proud of myself, to be honest! Besides, I have my friends and husband with me and....

"Sharon! You are bleeding!" My girlfriend looks at me in horror. I look down. There are big drops of blood on the table and now in my soup. Oh joy. I have a bloody nose! I go to grab the napkin. Tommy snatches it away, horrified that I might leave a napkin with blood on it. (I would have stolen it.)

"Then give me your sleeve! Or get the paper towel out of my pocket."

He manages to do that; I excuse myself and make a quick exit. The stares were knives in my newly brave heart. It wasn't enough that I presented as an alien, now I had blood all over my face. LOVELY.

I was so *humiliated*.

I got to my car and regrouped in private. What was happening?

Then it hit me. NOSE HAIR!!!!! Oh my God, *I had no nose hair!*

When the blood stopped, I took advantage of the privacy of my car and looked. Sure as you're born, those nostrils are as clear as a baby's bottom.

I can do the bald head. I can stand up proud and tall and do that. I can do no eyelashes or eyebrows. But I'm still not sure how to rock the blood all over my face. That may be out of my skill set.

The deal with losing one's nose hairs is that you no longer have a filter to keep allergens and whatever from going up your nose, you also have nothing to slow the departure *out* your nose. So, lots of times I just have a tiny little drip going on. Now I am sure that lots of people get used to this and have the dignity to constantly have a lovely little handkerchief in tow. I'm not that person. I'm like a kid – when there is a tiny trickle, I am a sleeve girl. Or the back of my hand until I can locate something more appropriate. When it happens a lot, which it has been lately, it kind of becomes the norm and you don't think about it too much. Most of the time it's not like you need to blow, and you don't because there is nothing holding this in to *warrant* a blow. Just drip…drip…drip.

Fair warning: It feels just like a bloody nose. And you get *used* to it. So when the lack of hairs fail to block something that *gives* you a bloody nose, you don't *think* it is a bloody nose, you *think* it's just more of the same bullshit, and when it starts happening there is a propensity to just wipe that drip off with the back of your hand. And possibly smear it all over your face. Not enough to be bald, which is quite noticeable on its own, now I get to look like some sort of *crime victim.*

"Are you going back in?"
"Never."
"I thought the plan was to have some fun with your friends."
"It was. I did."
"So you are saying that the family that kept staring at you from across the room, whom you do NOT know, is more important than having more fun with your friends?"

I hadn't looked at it like that, but it was a good point. I was saved by the bell, however. As I got out of the car, I saw them already on their way back. No doubt that my girlfriend got the part where a re-entry by me was highly unlikely. My husband was just happy enough to see me standing and not in a pool of blood. He got in the passenger seat and announced that I was driving.

OMG, I was driving us home! I could do it! My wings were back! I had some freedom and autonomy finally! I forgot all about my humiliation and reveled in yet another step toward having my life back.

17. JUST TWO MORE TO GO

Two more treatments to go. This should be a big "yeehaw" moment for me! It's been working great and it's not insurmountable – I feel crappy for a few days and then good for a couple weeks then repeat. I'm no longer half on my deathbed in excruciating pain. And it's almost over, so what the hell is my problem? Why am I feeling depressed?

Terminal has been pretty quiet and withdrawn as well, which I find unusual. Mind you, I have appreciated the sense (false, but whatever) of privacy, but I'm starting to get a little worried. So, I go rouse him and ask him how he is feeling.

"About the same as you."
"Do you know why? Because I don't understand what is going on with me at all. I worry that I am getting worse, that there is something else happening and I just don't know it."
He looks at me for a moment and gives me a small, sad little smile.
"That is because you have seen so much. That is just who you are, Sharon, and you know that the fear of something doesn't necessarily make it a reality. You're OK, kid."
"Then why am I so sad?"
"Because it is coming to a close. And if we finish the work we are doing together, you may have to say goodbye to some things that

have become a crutch for you."

I thought about this for several minutes. I'm still a little lost. And then it hit me like a ton of the weirdest bricks ever. It's saying goodbye to the *chemo*. Who the hell is afraid of THAT?

But I know why. The chemo got me out of a wheelchair and out of pain. The chemo was my sword. With it I felt that I was in some sort of control and finally able to fight back. The chemo kept me alive! Now it is almost done. I was losing my sword and I felt at the mercy of the enemy. Helpless, again. Scared, again.

"So now what? Do I just go have a couple good months and then it's over? What am I supposed to do? It feels like getting the original diagnosis all over again. Except that time, I knew. Now I don't know."
"I think they call that faith, Sharon. You need to have a little faith in yourself, even if 'yourself' feels so new and unsettled. You have only gotten stronger, even if you don't see it in anything but its physical manifestation right now. Chemo helped with that, but you are underestimating your own mind and where you have come."

It's Fear of the Unknown again. I can see that now. Like learning to walk without a crutch.

"It's OK to be scared and a little sad. You have been very stoic and brave. A few tears and a little sadness will not take away your basic personality. You won't crash completely. It's not in your make-up. You love life too much. You will get bored with being sad before you go under, my friend, trust me on that. It's OK to cry."

He looked out of one of his pristine windows. It was blank. Just swirling mist. No shape could be made out. Just Nothing. I stared at it too. He reached over and took my hand.

"Termy? Why are YOU so sad?"
He didn't speak for a long time. Then he said, "Because I've grown to love you. When you are sad, I am sad."

SUDDENLY TERMINAL

"I don't know what to say. I don't understand."
"I get lonely. I'm like the guy who comes bearing gifts that no one opens or just throws away. You did what your son taught you to do all those many years ago. And I am grateful."

I hadn't thought about that in *years*. But it is indelibly etched in my brain and probably one of my most life-defining moments. So, I'm going to share it:

I was in my mid-30s, newly divorced and raising my two sons on my own. And, like most young women in that situation, looking for love in all the wrong places. I have never been a fan of organized religion, but my belief in God and my relationship with God is very steadfast. My point is that I had never taken my children to church. One day Brandon, who was seven, came outside and found me crying in the garden. He asked me what was wrong and I told him that I was just sad because I couldn't meet a nice man.

Understand that my youngest child is no ordinary kid. He then rolls his eyes, gives an exasperated sigh, leans against the fence and says to me, "Mom? Do you know what your problem is?" Trying not to laugh at his little exaggerated "parental moment," I responded in the negative. "You are impatient and you don't have any faith."

I wasn't ready for *this*, I assure you. I asked for some clarification. "Well, Mom. You asked God for something and he gave you a big beautiful wrapped-up present. You got all excited and opened it. But all you found there was dirt. And you were mad and threw it away. You do this all the time. You have to have some *faith*, Mom. You have to dig through the box of dirt and find the diamond you asked for in the middle." I was gob smacked, but I have tried to live my life by that. And, I can clearly see now that that included Terminal. The trick is that you have to throw out a lot of the dirt to *find* the diamond. Terminal has helped me with that in spades.
I realized I was *grateful* then. Still not sure what I asked for, but I am grateful for the sorting and I trust that there was a reason. I may

not *know* the reason this has happened, but I have faith it happened for a reason.

I squeezed Terminal's hand as he continued to stare out the window. I stared too, into the mist. We don't know what is coming, but I will handle it.

"Thanks," I whispered.
"You too."

18. CHEMO NUMBER FIVE

I've been bringing food to the infusion room the last couple of times for everybody. This time I decided to do something besides just soup. I decided to make pretty little tea sandwiches to go along with it.

Lots of prep work the day before and off I go to chemo, armed and dangerous with all my food.

So much *fun!* I was in the little "kitchen in the back," with Mr. Stick (my IV dude) just putting these pretty little topless sandwiches together. I got tired in the middle of it, and found out that it was the Benadryl drip, so sandwich-making was cut short. After a brief nap, I was back in action, with Kerrylea's help, and it all went out on a beautiful cart to the staff.

This says a lot for my medical team, if you stop and think about it. No way in hell would you be allowed to just wander in the back room and do your own thing anywhere else. Mind you, she popped in every few minutes to check on me, but they were 100% behind me living my life and being who I am. And the fact that "who I am" is someone who really likes to feed people, doesn't exactly hurt.

I got it done and went back to Benadryl drip number two.

One of the other women in the room was really not doing well. The doctor came out and talked to her for a minute. Then he came over and said something to me that I thought was a compliment about lunch and I duly went back to sleep.

It was a good day.

The next day I thought I was going to have more steroid-juice energy than I did, but I decided that I wanted to know more about the insurance company denial of my medical care. (My brain was coming back a bit). I had a call in to my doctor, who called back that evening. I asked him about all of that. He told me that they would likely come back at me with the fact that I had metastatic cancer and I was going to die anyway so why spend $16K on shots? He said he told them that I was healthy, young (wow – don't hear that much at my age! I should have asked for that in writing!) and am very committed to getting better. "And I was right! 442!!!"

It took me a minute. I had no *idea* I had metastatic cancer. Wasn't sure what that meant, exactly, just that it is an out-of-control cancer that invades your entire being. Well, I guess I knew that part, but I didn't know it had *that* scary name. Then 442 hit me.

"What 442?"

"Your numbers. Your cancer markers are down to 442. You *did* it! I told you this *yesterday*."

I was reeling. It was comedown day after chemo, and I was definitely *not* on my game.

"I thought they were 3200."

"Yes, after your *third* chemo. I got the results from your *fourth* chemo yesterday: 442. *I told you this!*"

Now maybe he told me this during my Benadryl bag, but even then, I am pretty sure I would remember *this*.

"What, *exactly* did you tell me, Doc?"

"I said, 'Way to turn the Titanic around, woman!'"

Holy shit – I thought he was talking about LUNCH! After I had him reaffirm this 25 times, I dragged myself upstairs to tell Tommy. I was pretty flat in my delivery due to my physical state, but boy howdy – you better believe there were *fireworks* going off inside me.

I love my husband. I love my husband. I *love* my husband. But SOMETIMES I just want to smack him upside the head. This was one of those times.

"Well, that's *great* honey, but don't get *too* excited; this might be just like being on a diet. You know, it could be like the last ten pounds – they can be the hardest to lose!"

I just stared at him with the evilest glare I could conjure up.

"First off, *do not pee on my happy.* Don't you DARE PEE ON MY HAPPY! Secondly, what in the hell would *you* know about *dieting*? Your idea of a diet is eating three celery sticks and two carrot sticks before you polish off a bag of *Fritos!*"

I duly marched off to my couch-nest after that. But I knew, I *knew* that he didn't want to get his hopes up, nor mine. But seriously, watching one season of "The Biggest Loser" does not make him an oncologist. But he *is* right: *We don't know for sure.*

"Do you think YOU know? I think you do."
"Yep. I do. Thanks, Termy."

"No problem kiddo. Have a good night. Hang in there this week."
"Lifetime Movies – here I come!" And with a wane smile I went to
sleep.

Coming back out of these things is a trip. In a way it is like having
the flu; you slowly start to feel better and then you gradually are
OK. With this I slowly start to come around after three days, but
by day seven – *look out*. I swear it is like going from zero to sixty
in five seconds. A switch gets flipped and BAM! I'm back *full
throttle*.

While I had spent the week lolling about like some sort of seal
basking in the sun, reveling in the number 442, now I was wide
awake and facing chemo six.

We haven't even counted chemo five yet and I did the math – I
was assassinating about 2500 markers a month. With only 442 to
go, I should be at 0 easily, with 2000 to spare. (Tommy's analysis
aside, of course). I call, and the nurses tell me that I do, indeed,
have to do the last chemo. When I ask why, they tell me that is
because of hidden cells and little things of that sort. OK, that
makes sense. HOWEVER, 2000 markers should cover this,
right? It's not like doing an extra-credit essay on your English
test. Do I get to store these somewhere so if and when the cancer
comes back, I can say, "Wait! I got this! Hang on!" then run down
to the vault to get my Get-Out-of-Cancer-Free card and bring it
back? Somehow, I don't think so.

I don't profess to be an oncologist and I will do what he tells me to
do. I trust him implicitly. But this time, I need a good answer to the
question.

While the answer wasn't what I had hoped for, it was what I
expected: chemo 6, here I come. There may be one renegade little
asshole cell floating around in there, so we have to zap his butt!
Meanwhile I'm waiting, nervous as a feral cat, to hear the results
from my blood test. What are my new markers? I "think" they are
zero – I "feel" like the cancer is gone. What if I'm *wrong*? I might

be wrong. Seeing as I have another treatment to go, it isn't that worrisome – I have another shot at it.

Along comes the day of waiting for the results. I was on edge all day; then I got *the* call.

I was at 61. One would THINK that this would have me ecstatic. But *nooooo*. I wanted 0 (I'm never going to see zero, btw. This is *metastatic* cancer - the doc is just trying to get me under 30). But Superwoman wanted ZERO. I got 61 instead.

I burst into tears, ripped off my Superwoman cape and used it to blow my nose. A lot. No amount of encouragement, reasoning, or telling me how fantastic this is from my family was going to work. I was a spoiled, petulant, two-year-old and I simply wasn't havin' it. *They* were thrilled but I was falling apart. I took off my leotard with the big "S" on it and shredded it. The Brave Little Camper had come to an abrupt halt.

Everyone was telling me that I should be happy - I shouldn't be feeling the way I was. Certainly not sobbing in disappointment. Deep down I saw the logic there, but I was *way* past logic at that moment. Logic didn't matter. Ego mattered, I guess. I had this! I was going to beat this! I was at ZERO! I KNEW IT!

I was *wrong*. That is all I got out of the words "sixty-one" - I was *wrong*.

Tommy had to go back to work, Rachel was smart enough to realize that I would likely start looking for a target and left, so Brandon got stuck with me.

They were all bewildered as to why, exactly, I was crying over something that was downright amazing news. To be honest, so was I. My poor son just sat in front of me, holding my hands, both physically and mentally, while I tried to sort it out in my head. I was feeling *relief*. Well disguised, admittedly, but that is what it was. I've known all along that this cancer was going to kill me, but

I never looked down. There was a vast hole beneath me and I knew, intuitively, that if I fell into that hole of depression I would *never* get out. It was too deep. It was like a bottomless well. I had marched on bravely, only focusing on what I needed to do. I could not look at tomorrow, never mind have *hope* for it. I couldn't look at yesterday either. Yesterday and how close I came to dying was something that I am not sure I will ever be able to look at, truth be told. Yesterday was *gone* and today, *today* felt hopeful, admittedly, but also very untrustworthy. I simply crashed in the middle of it. I had been through so much! So much terror, looking at the end of my life all of a sudden. Unexpectedly. The proverbial rug had been YANKED out from under me. What the fuck? I should have *known*! I should have caught this! I should have, should have, should have...sobbing uncontrollably. What did I put my family through? Their love for me imprisoned them. Their lives got shut down alongside mine. I looked at my son and apologized, over and over again. I know he thought that I was apologizing for falling apart, but I wasn't. I was apologizing for every little "mom" thing I had ever done, for not being perfect enough to have my shit together and, most of all, for becoming so damn *needy* that I couldn't get to the bathroom in time. For all he had been put through, for all I *put* him through. It all came rushing in at once. I felt sorry for him, for Tommy, but mostly for *myself.* I felt sorry for my little self. Little Sharon, who never saw this coming and did the one thing she feared the most - took my loved ones hostage because of the fact that they love me. I cried *so hard.* He kept holding my hands (except for Kleenex time) and he listened, *really* listened to me. He cried, too.

It was good for me. And I think it was good for Brandon. There is a big difference between knowing you are going to die "someday because we all are," and knowing that you are going to die pretty soon and *why*. Things become more precious to you. A minute to share something like that with my youngest child, who feels it as intensely as I do, is one of those precious things.

Brandon managed to get me in the house and turn me over to Tommy who kept trying to get me to grasp the whole "percentages" thing until I finally fell asleep.

I woke up very early and when I did, I was still sad. It wasn't until I walked into my studio that what they had been trying to tell me hit me. I had a *choice*. Again. I could keep feeling sorry for myself or I could be happy and carry on with the life I still had. I've never been the kind of person who engages in self-pity for long. It's flat out *boring*.

I snapped out of it then. I'm alive.

61 isn't a bad number. I'm 61 years old! And I'm going to get to see 62! I'm ready to plan my 62nd birthday now!

And dammit! One more chemo or not, zero or *not* (I learned later *nobody* has zero), I *did* turn the Titanic around and I am headed straight for the Remission Iceberg instead.

"NO! Icebergs are NOT your friend! Take the damn thing to the BOAT TERMINAL!"

19. CHEMO BRAIN

I've heard the term from people whom I have watched go through this, but I kinda thought of it being similar to "artistic license"; in other words, not a real thing.

Ooooohh, was I ever wrong about THAT one! It's *very* weird. In the beginning I didn't notice it much because I was so damn out of it anyway that I just figured it was part and parcel of the cancer, but after I started to see the cancer part go away, well....

The first thing I noticed was that I kept thinking that things were real, but bizarre as hell and then realized that I had fallen asleep for a minute and was still in a dream state. OK, I got that. I did a lot of couch time during this and would doze off from time to time.

Sometimes I would wake up and everything was in two colors – yellow and black. At first, I thought our TV was screwy, but learned that a few blinks brought me back to Technicolor.

Once I started feeling better and had *part* of my mental capacity back, it started to go like this: Did I dream that or did that *actually* happen? If something obscure like a dragon or a tornado was involved, I knew it was a dream hangover, but usually it was more along the lines of people having done or said this or that. That was very confusing. And frustrating for those around me when I got it wrong, so I tended to just keep my mouth shut about it.

"Have you ever dreamt about a dragon?"
"No, that's just creative license in order to illustrate a point."
"I see. So that's a lie, essentially"
"Well.... I consider it my imagination. Which, I might point out, you are a part of as well."
"Good point. Does that make me a dragon?" He eyeballs me mischievously and begins a very poor imitation of a dragon. I'm just glad he can't work a lighter.
"I'm being serious, Terminal. Was I losing my mind? AM I losing my mind?"
"Not in the way you are thinking. Both your body and your mind are fighting for your life and the veil between the realities got lifted a bit. This may come as a shock to you, but even YOUR brain can't handle everything all at once. Chemo is a drug. Remember that. You are on drugs!" He starts laughing.
"Yeah, but I never dropped acid."
"Have you forgotten the great mushroom OD of 1979?"
I looked at him in absolute horror, "Yes! I remember that! Dear God, don't tell me that is what chemo is going to do to me! That was seriously NOT funny, and I damn near lost my mind that night."

Seeing the absolute terror in my eyes, he assured me that it was not like *that* and that I'm not 19 anymore and, while this is unnerving, it really isn't scary.

Easy for *him* to say!

Assurances aside, Terminal cannot resist a good song. And now we are on the Jefferson Airplane.

"One pill makes you larger and the other one makes you small, and the ones that mother gives you, don't do anything at all........ Remember what the dormouse said!... Feed your head! Feed your head!!"

Such a *special* moment.

The Chemo Brain got better as I did, but it is still here and still happening. And it is very, very weird when it does. Someone will attempt to explain the simplest thing to me and I just cannot grasp it. Sometimes I catch myself, like the other day, with something in each of my hands and needing to pick up my garden clippers. I stand there totally *stumped* on how to do that.

"Set something down, oh Bright One. You are not an octopus; you only have two hands."

YES! *That's the ticket!* I look at the things in my hands and, lo and behold, they *belong* where I am standing. Good gravy.

The next noteworthy episode was downright embarrassing.

I've lost a lot of weight and, on account of that, two of my rings don't fit anymore and I am in danger of losing them. I take them to a jeweler to be resized. I'm not a big jewelry person but these rings mean a lot to me. I wear four. On my left hand, I wear my wedding ring and on my little finger I wear my mother's wedding ring. On my right hand, I wear the birthstone ring I got on my 16th birthday from my mom (has quite a history behind it, actually) and a duplicate ring that was my best friend's birthstone ring (another story behind it: I had it made for her; she passed from brain cancer a few years ago). So, you can see that these rings *really* matter. A couple of weeks later they called me and told me to come get my rings. I'm super excited. It may sound silly, but I felt naked without them. The jeweler did a beautiful job and I put them on. They fit perfectly and they are like shining beacons of light on my hands and…. my other two are downright *filthy*. I point this out and my jeweler takes them from me to clean them. I'm shocked how easy they are to get off, actually. I take a mental note of that. That, right there, was the last "mental" note I seemed to take for the rest of the day. I paid my bill and was going to go to my friend's pub to wait for the other rings to be cleaned. I turned and took seven steps towards the door and looked at my hands.

SUDDENLY TERMINAL

Oh My God!!! I looked in horror, I was missing two rings? My birthstone and my wedding ring were *gone*!? What happened? Dear God, what happened? I calmed down and managed to remember I had them on when I was at the counter. Three minutes and seven steps ago.

The highly alarmed jeweler reminded me that they were in the machine being cleaned.

I've never been so happy for my bald head. *Very* embarrassed, I laughingly pointed at said head and said, "Chemo brain, sorry!" There were several episodes after that, things like wondering how to put the key in my ignition and where the keys are, only to come back to the planet and remember I push a button to start my car and there *are no keys*. It is a wonder I made it home.

And….. somebody found a new song!
"They are coming to take me away ho ho, hee hee, ha ha, to the funny farm where life is beautiful all the time…"

I wondered if one could go to jail for killing an imaginary asshole.

20. CHEMO NUMBER SIX

I was pretty off-kilter over this one. I'm really not sure why. I know I was "disappointed" in my marker count from number five, but I, once again, just put my head down, set my shoulders straight, and soldiered on.

Tommy had made a beautiful chocolate mousse cake with raspberry sauce for the occasion, which I brought in, and then found my seat. I've never seen the infusion room so busy. The nurses were already in a state with some sort of computer hell, and there were people *everywhere*. One man, who I have seen before, was in a bad way, obviously very sick. And another poor woman, Mexican and not English speaking, was in *hell*. Scared half to death, new port not working, veins failing, and in terrible pain with each re-stab (and these nurses are *good*). While Rosa speaks a fair bit of Spanish (thank God), the woman did not really understand and was *terrified*. She kept looking over at me, her eyes very reminiscent of one of those poor animals on that horrible Save the Animals commercial. Eventually, I couldn't take it anymore and went over to her where I could put my hand on her, wishing that I knew the Spanish word for "breathe." I had to settle for an encouraging smile and "It's OK."

Her terror hit straight home with me. I know why she had zeroed in on me. I was up, I was around, I had clearly done this already and was seemingly all right. I was *hope*. Finally, they got her sorted and she was able to go to sleep for a bit (or they put her to sleep – they can *do* that!) When she woke up, I was able to spend a bit of time with her, using my broken Spanish. We laughed a bit and she was able to tell me about her situation.

When I returned to my seat, I thought a lot about this; about how *far* I've come. Four months ago that was *me* in that chair. Scared, confused, and in pain. I was on a huge leap of faith, grasping at a single, solitary thread. If this didn't work, I was going to die.

I was going to die last month, actually. Wow.

"Yep. You be on borrowed time, sista!"
"Good morning Terminal. Sleep late?"
"I've been in meetings."
"Meetings? Dare I ask who you are having meetings with?"
"Hypochondria, Self-Pity, Compassion, among others, and The Boss, of course. Over Active Imagination was summoned, but said he was busy with you this weekend."
"I'll say. The Boss is Death, right?"
"That's what you call him. He prefers 'The Boss'. Big Springsteen fan. I call him El Jefe. He's not a big fan of that, however."
"I bet he isn't." Typical Terminal. Always the smart ass. *"This makes me nervous."*
"Oh for chrissakes, Sharon – EVERYTHING makes you nervous. We have meetings sometimes. Get over it."
"Well, what was THIS meeting about?"
"It's pretty much a progress report."
"Dammit, Terminal! If you don't elaborate, I swear I am going to lock you in your room for a month and completely disallow ANY form of music."

With that, the sarcastic little fuck breaks into the old Virginia Slims' ad, "You've Come a Long Way Baby!"

I want to throttle him. "Dammit, Terminal! Answer my question –
WHAT WAS THE MEETING ABOUT?!"
Now folding his arms and glowering at me, "THAT is what it was
about, you idiot!"
I say nothing.
"The Boss wanted to know where we all were with the matter. A
status report on the project."
"So now I am a 'project'? Lovely. Maybe we should start another
reality TV show and call it 'Project Dawson.' To hell with 'Project
Runway.'"'
"And this is why Sarcasm didn't have to be there. He said you
have maintained his position well and your numbers were coming
up in his department. Obviously, he has done a good job with you
over the years."
"Well, you are no slouch in the sarcasm department yourself." He
took a bow if only to illustrate the point. I laughed.
"Compassion and Empathy said that they were worried a bit at
first when you locked them in their rooms and wouldn't even look
at either of them, but I told them you just needed a break from
them. And since there was no room for them when I first got here,
they went to some tropical place. The Boss did tell them to keep an
eye on you because you do have a propensity to overdo it. But they
assured him that Tommy seems to have kept you in check pretty
well – remember the homeless guy, John? The one you took out to
lunch a couple of times and you thought about bringing him home
but you didn't because of Tommy? That was a huge sigh of relief
for those guys."
"Back into the archives, I see."
"Research, baby! I told you it's a big part of the job."
"Hmmm. I think 'Nosey' would be more apropos."
"Whatever. As I was saying, Balance was there and said he still
has his hands full. Self-pity was there and said you guys had a
banner day on Friday, but that it was long overdue. He had been
looking pretty shoddy up until then, I must say. You haven't let him
out much. And that's OK. He likes being small, but sometimes you
have to feed him for your own sake. Gratitude is your best weapon,
and I must say, she is an Amazon Woman. She has taught you to be
a glass-is-half-full kind of girl. She's done well. Some people call

her 'Faith.'"
I thought Optimism might work, but Faith is much prettier.
He continued, "Overactive Imagination said that things were
going OK. This is his week off as Hypochondria tends to take the
forefront (and is very excited, btw) but that you have been putting
him to good use throughout (for the most part) and, frankly he is
proud of you."
I digested this for a minute. "And the Boss?" I was scared to ask.
"He is more about receiving our reports than he is on stating his
opinions. He pretty much takes it all into consideration."
"OK. What was YOUR report?"
"Let's talk about that later. You are tired. Get some sleep".

I didn't argue. Apparently during my musings, they had changed
my IV to Sleepy Bag IV, and I went *out.*

When I woke up, I saw a couple coming in that I had seen a few
times before. He was a patient -- a very nice man – and his wife
was absolutely delightful. I had met them at the beginning and he
was in as much pain as I. When they came in this time *he* still was.
I'm across the room from them, but it's a small room. The doctor
came in to talk to them. The nurse was standing there. Terminal
told me to listen. (Normally we try to ignore out of privacy, even
though we can hear if we want to.) The doctor had good news for
them. He had come in with markers of 700+ and was now down to
300+ and had beat it down 50%. The nurse was locked right into
my eyes.

All I could think about was what a fucking, naive, spoiled rotten
brat I had been. Good God!. I know that cancer and treatment are
radically different for everyone, but I didn't know what that meant
in reality. By the time my markers had come down to where he
started, I was out of my wheelchair, out of pain and joining the
gym, for chrissakes! And here he was, fighting for every single
marker he could get off, suffering *still*. And here I was feeling like
a million bucks compared to where I was, crying over 61 lousy
markers because the spoiled little princess that I am wanted less
than *that*.

I was so *ashamed* of myself. Instead of extreme gratitude, I had thrown a full-blown hissy fit. Few things in my life have been, or ever will be, as humbling as that was.

If *that* wasn't enough, there was a woman in the chair next to me whom I had never seen before. She was very friendly and wanted to chat. She told me that she was "finally" able to resume her chemo treatments.

When I had started on this path, my doctor told me that very few women made it past the third or fourth chemo and he really, *really* wanted me to get through at least four. In my dazed and stunned state, I had thought he meant that it was just so horrible that they couldn't take it anymore and quit.

After my first one, when the stupid insurance company denied me a shot and my white blood cells went down to a whopping 25 cells, I figured that was it; white blood cells. At my last appointment I asked him about that. He told me that was *not* it, pointing out that they can boost the white blood cells (stupid insurance companies not withstanding); it is because of the RED blood cells and their platelets. (I think it is palettes. Little plates, I guess.) *That* they can't fix, your body has to do that and if they fall too low, you will die. But, he tells me that I don't have to worry about that. As a matter of fact, he has never seen anything quite like this. At that point he spins the computer screen around with a dramatic flourish. (He has done this before. It's fun for him.) Now I am looking at my "chart" with rows of numbers that I don't begin to understand. He shows me my red count. Started around 11 and has steadily gone up to 14. Wow! Look at THAT! I have no idea what this means. *None whatsoever.* Remembering that I am about as far away from a medical degree as a human can get, he explains: I make a lot of blood. A hell of a lot of blood. I should donate blood, as a matter of fact. He's all aglow over this. I'm happy because he is happy. Go little red blood cells, go! But I seriously didn't get it.

Then comes the woman in the chair next to me. The reason she was forced to quit her treatments was her red count. She had taken time off hoping they would multiply faster than her cancer cells so she could resume. Dear God.

While we chatted about her rock-star shoes and varying other things, internally I was melting, just like the Wicked Witch of the West and *sure* I was just about as horrible. I've been so very, very lucky.

It's amazing what you can learn about yourself when you listen to others.

Terminal did something then, that he's never done before. He manifested in my chair next to me and wrapped his arms around me. *"Now you know what I told The Boss."*

I fell asleep.

When I was done (early this time!) Tommy came to pick me up and I watched everyone fall at his feet over the cake and him deservedly beaming away over the whole thing. I was surprisingly tired. I know they gave me some steroids, but apparently, they didn't have the same effect as in the past. I was kind of disappointed, to be honest. That stuff is great! I might babble on and drive everyone around me clinically *insane*, but hell! I felt GOOD, baby, and when you feel like shit all the time, a day of feeling GOOD is worth the price of admission! (Well, maybe not.) The fallout on this one was not so much fun. I had to go up for my white cell shot the next day and could barely stay awake. I nearly fell asleep during the shot. But I managed to rally a bit for Tommy's birthday. Then I completely crashed.

The next day was hard, but it always is. Last time the neuropathy was barely there. This time it was back in *spades*. Thursday it was clear up to my knees and I couldn't walk with any kind of confidence, sure I was going straight down. I hurt. I was more nauseous than I had ever been. I was sure the neuropathy had settled in and was here to stay! My pee was the wrong color. What the hell was happening?

I can see why Hypochondria had been looking forward to this week. He's had a *field* day with me. While I knew, intellectually, that it was "over," emotionally I was terrified and didn't feel like it was over at all. How could I get away so easily? Why *me*? Did I deserve this? No. I don't deserve this anymore than anyone else. And there I was again, waiting for yet another shoe to drop.

"Oh, Good Gravy, Woman! Would you STOP already?"
"These are questions worth asking, Terminal."

"Maybe they are. But you absolutely cannot know the answers to 'why.' You can't. I don't even know those answers. Just get through the week. Get through the chemo brain. Revisit this next week, OK?"

He sounded tired and sad. Nothing snarky, no sarcasm, just sad.

"You OK, Term?"
"Yeah. I'm fine. Just got a lot on my mind."

Four months ago, I would have moved in on him like a hyena on a weakened animal. But not now. I have changed. Our *relationship* has changed. We have gotten to a place of understanding. Not an *agreement*, mind you, but an understanding of each other.

I went to bed and slept peacefully for the first time in a week.

21. WAKE UP DAY

4:15 AM. I'm awake. It's not that unusual, but there is no going back to sleep this time because it is the End of Constipation Day and the bowels are active.

The constipation is hell. I've discussed that. And while I look forward to it being *over*, I sure as hell don't look forward to the damn process. I've had it take up to 4 hours. I tell myself that this is the last time. I get up. Hey! No neuropathy. None last night, come to think of it. OK!

One hour and 15 minutes later, things are out of my body at last and….. *I'm a new woman*! Once again, it is like a light switch. But this time…..this time…..*this time* it is really and truly OVER! This time is the *last* time!

Like a rush of wind my mind and energy came back. And it hit me. I *did* it. It was *over*. While I may never have dreamed of a dragon, I sure as hell slew one. I cried tears of happiness; something I have not done in a very, very long time.

The reality is huge. I should have been dead at least a month ago. At one point I was extremely clear on this based on my own body, never mind what I was told. This was my last thread of hope. And it worked. By God, it *worked*.

I know it isn't a "forever" kind of gig, but it sure as hell is a "for now" kind of gig and I will take it for as long as I can get it. I've had a mind-blowing amount of support from my inner circle, from my community and a hell of a lot of "followers" that I don't know except for responses to my writing. All these people really prayed for me (OK, prayed, blessed, did little dances around a flower – whatever you need to call it, they *did* it).

I have after care – some sort of immunotherapy that I have to do every three weeks, but I can't take a pill....noooooo... this is the same stuff I have been getting alongside my chemo that I had the reaction from hell to, so I have to get it *slowly*. Meaning I will go in for IV drip every three weeks for the rest of my life. (This is God's idea of humor, by the way.) Takes an hour – no fallout from it, and only one hour instead of ten hours? *Not a problem.* Not a problem at *all*.

I know it will be back someday. But it won't be back *tomorrow*. Or next month.

I posted this on my social media page – that I finally pooped and was ready to celebrate, I guess. Dear God, never in my wildest dreams did I think I would be posting something of that nature. I guess my writing has evolved from Boyfriends to Bowel Movements. Who *knew*?

One thing that I kept getting online is about how "strong" I am and what a "warrior woman" I am. Being that I am the person who lives inside me, I'm not altogether sure that is true, but I know I am a brave little camper when push comes to shove.

"Until it comes to bicycles, or anything athletic, for that matter. Or really putting yourself out there with your art, or a myriad of things."
"Good morning. Did you come to rain on my parade?"
"No. Just want to make sure we have total visibility on this."
"What would I ever do without you?"

"I don't know." He sounded kind of sad. And he looks pretty much unkempt, which isn't like him. He usually employs that casual-but-I-worked-very-hard-at-it kind of look.

Before this happened to me to the level where Terminal actually came in, I believed that attitude was a big part of healing. Being strong, being a "warrior," never looking down, never giving up. I can't say I believe that has all that much to do with it now. Unless you *want* to die, you just do what you have to do to stay alive. It doesn't make you brave. Especially if you are like me and your cancer was at the end stage and clearly winning the game. Pain is a strong motivator, let me tell you! And when you begin to feel some reprieve from the pain on account of treatment, well…you keep going.

My nurse told me once when I was getting my shot that I was one of the bravest patients she had ever had. I just laughed and told her that I wasn't brave, I was *educated*. I didn't mean book-smart, I was educated in what this cancer could be like when it was allowed to run amok. Bravery has absolutely nothing to do with it. Bravery is not immunity. It does help you live, however.

I asked my doctor about this, actually. I just wanted to see if there were any studies about this in his field. Not surprisingly, he told me no. I knew that. Of course, one cannot measure the power of prayer and collective thinking – that will be beyond our scope of study until we die. *Then* we will know. But what he did tell me was impressive. He told me that while there are no scientific studies to indicate anything in regard to slowing the actual disease, he sees that it helps in quality of life. And that is the most important thing to him. To me as well. Even at my worst, I found beauty in a simple flower. I would look at it with new eyes, sometimes all day long, marveling at how it changed with the sun, and seeing its magnificent beauty like I had never seen it before. And it made me *happy*. I might be actively dying but, dammit, *I could still see the flower*.

This is what all of this has been about. Appreciating the little things. Living one's life to the fullest instead of waking up each day worrying about money. Instead of waking up each day worrying about approval or fighting with whatever inner demon that has plunged a knife into your gut and is now twisting it.

Why? Because we ARE ALL worthy of happiness. We think that we aren't worthy of it because we haven't achieved…*what*? What *exactly* did I think I had to achieve before I could be happy? Dear God.

Do you think you aren't worthy of a pretty flower? Can you even let yourself take the time to see it? That, right there, is quality of life. When Terminal rolls in and you find out that your life is going to end, you have two choices – embrace what you still have or go home. I chose to embrace it. For however long it was going to last, I wanted it. Every little sparkly sunray. Every dewdrop. *All of it.*

I learned a hell of a lot about myself and others through this. Terminal taught me so much. But I taught myself, too. He is, after all, only a part of me. He was my greatest fear. Now he is not. I wish I had figured this out before, but for me, I guess, I had to learn it the hard way.
Once again.

20. SAYING GOOD BYE TO TERMINAL

Terminal has just lugged a bag down the stairs, looking for all the world like a train wreck. He's very pale and clutching one of my skirts from college.

"What are you doing?"

He plops down on the last step and starts to cry.

"Dear God, what is wrong, Term?"
"Nothing."
"Oh for the love of all things holy, don't give me that bullshit. Clearly something is wrong."
"I am just closing up shop here." Sniff. *"That's all."*
"You're WHAT?"
"You are OK. My time here is over. I'm not sad about that, but I have grown to like you. You are my friend. You listen to me. That doesn't happen very much. But The Boss is pulling me off the job. I may be back, but I don't know. I hope not, but I am going to miss you very much. I know, that's bad. I want to be gone because I love you. But I kinda liked it here. I felt accepted here. I don't sing for just anybody, you know."

I can't even believe my reaction. In a weird way I have grown comfortable with him, too. Obviously, I don't want to be terminally ill anymore, but still… I've grown accustomed to his face. In a bizarre way I had gotten *used* to being terminally ill.

Now I have to get *used* to being *really* alive. And I have to do it on my own.

"Well, while I feel flattered that you don't sing for just anybody, I would encourage you to continue with that sort of discrimination."

This was my lame attempt at bringing sarcasm and humor into a conversation that had me highly unnerved. It didn't work. He just sat there; head drooped low

.

I was sad, too. Although it had only been six months, it felt like a lifetime. Probably because I had changed as much in those six months as I had in my *entire* lifetime.

"I'm sorry Term."
"Don't be. Please don't be. We don't really know; I may be back. I hope not. I hope El Jefe just does the job. Can I keep the skirt? Sometimes I have to go in as a female and it's a pretty cool skirt. I could show someone how to have some fun with it, maybe?"
He looks at me beseechingly.
"Of course you can! Take the whole damn closet for all I care. That stuff is long gone anyway!"
"Oh, I'm so glad you said that! So, are these OK, too?"
I look and he has the entirety of my huge silver bracelet collection stashed away. "Oh, you are such a little, thieving shit. Do you know that?" And we both laughed.

But for everything he took, he left plenty behind. That much I knew.

"Why now? Why do you have to leave now? I don't even know what my final numbers are!"'
"But I do. Love yourself, kiddo. I know I love you."

And just like that he was gone.

I whispered into the silent air around me, *"You really do have a great singing voice, Termy."*

The tears started then.

Relief came in and told me that it was normal, but I knew it was more than that; I had loved having him as a "guidance counselor," if you will. Now I had to do it on my own and I felt very shaky about that, to be honest.

All of a sudden, a moth-eaten, cobweb-ridden woman came in and put her arms around me. I had no idea who she was. She introduced herself to me as Self-Esteem.

The tears turned into uncontrollable sobs.

Two weeks later my number came in.

It was 14.

SUDDENLY TERMINAL

LETTER TO THE READER

This is my story. It's not my *whole* story, just my journey through my recovery. I have no idea when, or even if, the cancer will come back. They say it probably will, eventually. But in the interim I intend to live the life I have fought so hard for. Terminal is a figment of my imagination. That is partly the writer within, but I think in a lot of ways being able to compartmentalize this whole, sudden, and decidedly unexpected series of events into a *character*, an entity of its own, has enabled me to keep my sense of humor to a point and help to keep fear at bay. Many writers create characters that become very real to them. Some characters live on, some don't. We are not insane by *our* standards, but if you could hear what we hear, you may beg to differ.

If you, too, have found yourself in these shoes, I hope to God that this will help you. Maybe bring a smile to your face from time to time. Maybe some hope. But most of all, I hope that it will help you to live the life that you have right here and right now without focusing on what *may be* inevitable. Death *is* inevitable. The difference between you and that idiot who says, "Well, we will all die someday" is that you are looking at the tangible, and they are talking about the *intangible*. The gift for us, if we choose to see it in the middle of this terrifying and fucked up shit, is that we will truly be able to live each moment as if it is our last. We can learn to sort the chaff from the wheat and the beauty in the small things will intensify. Too much of our lives are spent postponing this.

I will die eventually and possibly not too many years from now. Frankly I would rather be hit by that proverbial bus, but most likely the cancer will take me. Until then I am going to live my life as fully as I can. I made my decision. That, at least, is my choice, and this is my journey.

When I first got the diagnosis, people would ask me what is on my bucket list. THIS was on my bucket list. To be able to write something and put it out there – to truly communicate – has been my life's dream. I think lots of people were expecting me to say something grandiose like "go see the pyramids" or something. (Hell, I could hardly ride in the damn car without hurting– screw the pyramids!) Nope. I just wanted to *write*. And maybe someday see New York City; just to see a few museums, go out for fabulous food and wear fun and sexy clothes in shoes I can't walk in! LOL

Thank you so very, *very* much for reading my little book.

It's a dream come true.

Sharon

Made in USA - North Chelmsford, MA
1309285_9798432157201
03.23.2022 0955